Special Care Dentistry

Editor

STEPHANIE M. MUNZ

DENTAL CLINICS OF NORTH AMERICA

www.dental.theclinics.com

April 2022 • Volume 66 • Number 2

ELSEVIER

1600 John F. Kennedy Boulevard • Suite 1800 • Philadelphia, Pennsylvania, 19103-2899

http://www.dental.theclinics.com

DENTAL CLINICS OF NORTH AMERICA Volume 66, Number 2
April 2022 ISSN 0011-8532, ISBN: 978-0-323-91967-8

Editor: John Vassallo; j.vassallo@elsevier.com
Developmental Editor: Ann Gielou M. Posedio

Dental Clinics of North America (ISSN 0011-8532) is published quarterly by Elsevier Inc., 360 Park Avenue South, New York, NY 10010-1710. Months of issue are January, April, July, and October. Business and Editorial Offices: 1600 John F. Kennedy Boulevard, Suite 1800, Philadelphia, PA 19103-2899. Periodicals postage paid at New York, NY and additional mailing offices. Subscription prices are $323.00 per year (domestic individuals), $854.00 per year (domestic institutions), $100.00 per year (domestic students/residents), $377.00 per year (Canadian individuals), $863.00 per year (Canadian institutions), $100.00 per year (Canadian students/residents) $441.00 per year (international individuals), $863.00 per year (international institutions), and $200.00 per year (international students/residents). International air speed delivery is included in all *Clinics* subscription prices. All prices are subject to change without notice. **POSTMASTER:** Send address changes to *Dental Clinics of North America*, Elsevier Health Sciences Division, Subscription Customer Service, 3251 Riverport Lane, Maryland Heights, MO 63043. **Customer Service (orders, claims, online, change of address): Elsevier Health Sciences Division, Subscription Customer Service, 3251 Riverport Lane, Maryland Heights, MO 63043. Tel: 1-800-654-2452 (U.S. and Canada). Fax: 314-447-8029. E-mail: journalscustomerservice-usa@elsevier.com (for print support); journalsonlinesupport-usa@elsevier.com (for online support)**.

Reprints. For copies of 100 or more, of articles in this publication, please contact the Commercial Reprints Department, Elsevier Inc., 360 Park Avenue South, New York, NY 10010-1710. Tel.: 212-633-3874; Fax: 212-633-3820; E-mail: reprints@elsevier.com.

The Dental Clinics of North America is covered in *MEDLINE/PubMed (Index Medicus), Current Contents/Clinical Medicine, ISI/BIOMED* and *Clinahl*.

Contributors

EDITOR

STEPHANIE M. MUNZ, DDS, FSCD
Walter H. Swartz Professor of Integrated Special Care Dentistry, Clinical Associate
Professor and Associate Chair of Hospital Dentistry, Department of Oral and Maxillofacial
Surgery/Hospital Dentistry, University of Michigan School of Dentistry, Ann Arbor,
Michigan, USA

AUTHORS

AKIHIRO ANDO, DDS
Director, Ando Orofacial Pain and Oral Medicine Clinic, Visiting Associate Professor,
Showa University School of Dentistry, Tokyo, Japan

STEPHEN BEETSTRA, DDS, MHSA
Dental Program Director, Nisonger Center, Wexner Medical Center, Ohio State University
Dental School, Columbus, Ohio, USA

MARCIA S. CAMPOS, DDS, MSc, PhD
Clinical Associate Professor, Department of Cariology, Restorative Sciences and
Endodontics, University of Michigan School of Dentistry, Ann Arbor, Michigan, USA

BRETT CHIQUET, DDS, PhD
Associate Professor, Department of Pediatric Dentistry, UTHealth, The University of Texas
Health Science Center at Houston, School of Dentistry

RONALD ETTINGER, BDS, MDS, DDSc, DDSc(hc)
Professor Emeritus, Department of Prosthodontics, The University of Iowa College of
Dentistry and Dental Clinics, Iowa City, Iowa, USA

MARGHERITA FONTANA, DDS, PhD
Professor, Department of Cariology, Restorative Sciences and Endodontics, University of
Michigan School of Dentistry, Ann Arbor, Michigan, USA

CLIVE FRIEDMAN, BDS
Cert. Pediatric Dentistry/Diplomate, American Academy of Pediatric Dentistry; Clinical
Associate Professor, Schulich School of Medicine and Dentistry

BROOKE FUKUOKA, DMD, FSCD
Your Special Smiles PLLC-Owner Dentist, Family Health Services Idaho-FQHC Dentist,
Twin Falls, Idaho, USA

PHUU P. HAN, DDS, PhD
Former Clinical Associate Professor, Herman Ostrow School of Dentistry of USC, Los
Angeles, California, USA

LIZBETH HOLGUIN, DDS
Certified, American Board of Pediatric Dentistry., Division Chief of Pediatric/Hospital Dentistry, El Paso Children's Hospital

SCOTT E.I. HOWELL, DMD, MPH
Associate Professor, Director of Public Health Dentistry & Teledentistry, A.T. Still University, Arizona School of Dentistry and Oral Health, Mesa, Arizona, USA

LISA E. ITAYA, DDS
Associate Professor and Outcomes Assessment Liaison, University of the Pacific. Arthur A. Dugoni School of Dentistry, San Francisco, California, USA

RAY A. LYONS, DDS, DABSCD, FADPD
Adjunct Professor, Dental Hygiene and Residency Program, University of New Mexico

LEONARDO MARCHINI, DDS, MSD, PhD
Associate Professor, Department of Preventive and Community Dentistry, The University of Iowa College of Dentistry and Dental Clinics, Iowa City, Iowa, USA

KIMBERLY MARIE ESPINOZA, DDS, MPH
Clinical Associate Professor-Dental Pathway, Department of Oral Medicine, University of Washington, School of Dentistry, Seattle, Washington, USA

SEENA PATEL, DMD, MPH
Associate Professor, Director of Oral Medicine, Arizona School of Dentistry and Oral Health, Advanced Care Center, A.T. Still University, Mesa, Arizona, USA; Associate, Southwest Orofacial Group, Phoenix, Arizona, USA

STEVEN P. PERLMAN, DDS, MScD, DHL (Hon), DABSCD
Global Clinical Director and Founder, Special Olympics Special Smiles, Clinical Professor of Pediatric Dentistry, Boston University Goldman School of Dental Medicine, Adjunct Faculty Penn Dental Medicine

RICK RADER, MD
Adjunct Professor, Human Development, University of Tennessee at Chattanooga

ALISON SIGAL, B.H. Kin, DDS, MSc (Peds Dent), FRCD(C)
Founder and Pediatric Dentist, Little Bird Pediatric Dentistry

MICHAEL SIGAL, DDS, Dip Peds, MSc, FRCD(C)
Professor Emeritus Pediatric Dentistry, University of Toronto, Pediatric Dentist, Little Bird Pediatric Dentistry

H. BARRY WALDMAN, DDS, MPH, PhD
Distinguished Teaching Professor, Department of General Dentistry, School of Dental Medicine, Stony Brook University, New York, New York, USA

JESSICA WEBB, DDS, MSD, MA, MSRT
Affiliate Assistant Professor, Department of Pediatric Dentistry, University of Washington, Associate Program Director, Advanced Education in Pediatric Dentistry, Postdoctoral Residency Programs, NYU Langone Dental Medicine

ALLEN WONG, DDS, EdD, DABSCD
Professor and Director, AEGD Program, Director of Hospital Dentistry Program, University of the Pacific Arthur A. Dugoni School of Dentistry, San Francisco, California, USA

SAMUEL ZWETCHKENBAUM, DDS, MPH
Dental Director, Oral Health Program, Division of Community Health and Equity, Rhode Island Department of Health, Center for Preventive Services, Providence, Rhode Island, USA

Contents

> The objective of this article is to provide a summary of the current evidence-based recommendations for caries management in patients with special health care needs (SHCNs). Considerations regarding caries risk assessment and preventive measures are also discussed with the goal of helping clinicians to manage the caries disease process using a person-centered approach and risk-based interventions. Importantly, most of the evidence is still based on the general population, because the evidence for those with SHCNs is still limited.

> In March 2020, the World Health Organization declared a global public health emergency due to the spread of COVID-19, and medical and dental elective care was suspended, disproportionally affecting persons with special needs. As many of the special needs population live in a communal environment, they were at higher risk of being infected with and dying of COVID-19. Consequently, their access to medical and dental services was limited to emergency care. A method of reaching these populations evolved by the expansion of telehealth, including dentistry, to provide diagnosis, management, prevention, and provision of psychosocial support for patients.

> Teledentistry is a powerful tool for connecting oral health providers with patients who cannot easily visit a dental office, such as patients with special health care needs. Teledentistry is a skill that must be learned and this article will review key concepts that will allow providers to be better prepared to use it within their practices. These concepts include considerations for data collection and information that is necessary for a successful teledentistry visit. The authors also provide different examples of teledentistry in action, such as guided oral hygiene or dental screenings. Lastly, the authors review some unique challenges related to teledentistry and recommendations for overcoming those challenges.

Video content accompanies this article at http://www.dental. theclinics.com.

This article provides a brief overview of how the environment can affect behavior and that well-designed spaces can affect how patients handle stress. The application of the Snoezelen multisensory interactive calming strategies and devices that were installed in all facets of a community dental practice are described. These principles of creating a calming dental home improved behavior, cooperation, and satisfaction with care in persons with disabilities and reduced the need for sedation or general anesthesia. It is proposed that the creation of similar clinics with multisensory calming features could improve community access to dental care for persons with special needs.

Nonodontogenic orofacial pain exists, and diagnosis and management of those conditions can be challenging. This article highlights and discusses how to take a complete and systematic pain history and the important red flags to recognize in patients presenting with perplexing nonodontogenic orofacial pain. Cause and epidemiology, clinical presentation, clinical evaluation and diagnosis, and management options for common neuropathic pain conditions are included. Neuralgia and neuropathic pain conditions and red flags as secondary cause of orofacial pain are more common in older-aged patients.

People with special health care needs experience barriers to oral health care resulting in oral health inequities. This article outlines avenues for advocacy to better serve these populations and reduce oral health inequities. Concepts of cultural humility can aid in advocacy efforts and include critical self-reflection, addressing power imbalances in health care relationships, and advocacy for change that influences the social determinants of health. Developing cultural humility is a lifelong process that requires ongoing learning and action in reducing health inequities and barriers to health care.

Clinical dental treatment is the most exacting and demanding medical procedure that persons with special needs undergo on a regular basis throughout their lifetime. Dental treatment is surgical in nature, usually requiring controlled placement of sharpened instrumentation in intimate proximity to the face, airway, and highly vascularized and innervated oral tissues. Although approximately 90% of patients with special needs can and should be mainstreamed through any general dental practice, without significant behavioral guidance, techniques, or medical immobilization/protective stabilization, over the past years there has been a drastic shift toward pharmacologic management of these patients using various forms of sedation and general anesthesia.

Special Care Dentistry

DENTAL CLINICS OF NORTH AMERICA

SERIES OF RELATED INTEREST

Atlas of the Oral and Maxillofacial Surgery Clinics

Oral and Maxillofacial Surgery Clinics

THE CLINICS ARE AVAILABLE ONLINE!
Access your subscription at:
www.theclinics.com

Preface

Now Is the Time for Special Care Dentistry

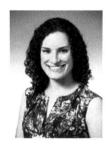

Stephanie M. Munz, DDS, FSCD
Editor

I am excited to share this emerging issue on "Special Care Dentistry" and make an honorable note of thanks and admiration to my predecessor and late editor, Dr Burton S. Wasserman, who paved the way with two issues in 2009 and 2016, on this important area of the oral health profession. It is with much enthusiasm these topics were proposed and vetted with the guidance of Mr John Vassallo, the editor of *Dental Clinics of North America*, and Ms Ann Gielou Posedio, the developmental editor, during what the profession will note to be one of the most catalyzing and evolving periods of our profession. The topics were selected to represent the breadth of patient management areas of expertise, to include the diversity of patient populations as well as the essentials of preventive and restorative care, and even innovative care delivery models in virtual health that were sparked and encouraged by the COVID-19 global pandemic. I thank the contributing authors for their dedication to the topics despite the obvious challenges.

This is a pinnacle time in special care dentistry. Educators in the dental profession collectively recognize the importance of training future oral health care providers to serve these vulnerable populations. The Special Care Dentistry Association (SCDA) has taken on two such initiatives to request for approval by the Commission on Dental Accreditation for advanced training programs in geriatric dental medicine (initiated in 2019) and special needs dentistry (initiated in 2021), which were sparked by resolutions passed by the American Dental Association House of Delegates and with leadership by the Council on Dental Education and Licensure. Advocates in the profession appreciate how critical it will be to have an equipped workforce for the care of persons with special health care needs (SHCNs) across the lifespan. This will include training the present workforce through various avenues to manage patients with increasing health and risk complexity across a variety of practice settings. Learners are also excited to gain the knowledge, skills, attitudes, and practice behaviors to

Dent Clin N Am 66 (2022) xi–xii
https://doi.org/10.1016/j.cden.2022.01.008
0011-8532/22/© 2022 Published by Elsevier Inc.

dental.theclinics.com

manage patients with SHCNs, so much so that training programs are now focused to respond to their trainees' energy and forward-thinking.

Meanwhile, three postgraduate training pathways with close connections to special care dentistry have each received dental specialty recognition in the United States, namely Dental Anesthesiology (adopted March 2019), Oral Medicine (adopted September 2020), and Orofacial Pain (adopted September 2020). Both SCDA and the American Academy of Developmental Medicine and Dentistry (AADMD) have partnered on initiatives to better understand and unravel the barriers to care for patients with SHCNs, and AADMD continues the superb advocacy and interprofessional education and collaboration efforts for which the organization is well known. Resources and reimbursement for vulnerable populations are continued topics of importance for the future. Across the profession, the trend is a zoomed-in focus on oral health topics related to persons with SHCNs. It is a fine time to be involved and invigorated in special care dentistry! I am forever grateful for the opportunity to be editor of this special issue.

Stephanie M. Munz, DDS, FSCD
Department of Oral & Maxillofacial Surgery/Hospital Dentistry
University of Michigan School of Dentistry and Michigan Medicine
Towsley Center G1210
1515 East Hospital Drive, Ann Arbor
MI 48109-5222, USA

E-mail address:
smmunz@umich.edu

Caries Management in Special Care Dentistry

Marcia S. Campos, DDS, MSc, PhD[a],*, Margherita Fontana, DDS, PhD[b]

KEYWORDS

- Dental caries • Risk assessment • Caries management • Special health care needs

KEY POINTS

- Lack of evidence regarding caries management in patients with special health care needs (SHCNs), variability of patients and their conditions, and general high-caries-risk patterns demand personalized care.
- Clinicians should apply caries risk assessment tools to better guide their therapeutic approach, inform prognosis, and determine preventive strategies. Caries risk should be reassessed over time to avoid disease progression.
- High-quality evidence shows sealants and fluoride toothpaste are able to prevent and arrest caries lesions in children, adolescents, and adults. Use of high-concentration fluoride toothpaste, topical application of silver diamine fluoride, fluoride varnish, and chlorhexidine varnishes is recommended as nonrestorative treatments for caries lesions that can be applied in patients with SHCNs.
- After assessing caries risk, the key is to focus on increasing prevention while decreasing risk factors. Diet control and reduction of sugar frequency are crucial, as well as supervised oral hygiene practices to help control plaque.
- When possible, minimally invasive procedures, such as atraumatic restorative treatment technique, should be applied to delay the restorative cycle, prolonging tooth survival. When restorative treatment is necessary, selective caries removal using hand excavators is recommended.

INTRODUCTION

Dental caries is a multifactorial and noncommunicable disease, which, despite advances in research and preventive approaches, remains a major public health problem that affects multiple populations at all ages.[1,2] It has been suggested that patients with special health care needs (SHCNs) generally present an increased risk for developing dental caries, although the literature provides sparse and conflicting data on this

---

[a] Department of Cariology, Restorative Sciences and Endodontics, University of Michigan School of Dentistry, 1011 North University, Room 3169, Ann Arbor, MI 48109, USA;
[b] Department of Cariology, Restorative Sciences and Endodontics, University of Michigan School of Dentistry, 1011 North University, Room 2303, Ann Arbor, MI 48109, USA
* Corresponding author.
E-mail address: mscampos@umich.edu

Dent Clin N Am 66 (2022) 169–179
https://doi.org/10.1016/j.cden.2021.12.003

subject. These patients often show higher prevalence of active and untreated caries lesions, difficulties to access care, and difficulties to accomplish good oral hygiene, leading to unmet dental needs.[3–6] Perhaps, even more than the general population, they are impacted by socioeconomic, demographic, motor skills, behavioral, and psychological factors representing a challenge for clinicians, family, and caregivers.[3–6] In addition, the variety of conditions and severity of disabilities make the creation of a protocol for the entire spectrum of these patients more difficult. This article generalizes the discussion about them simply based on how unique they are. With that in mind, person-centered care approaches have been emerging as the future of the health care system,[7] and, for this reason, tools for caries assessment that can be used interprofessionally should be developed, as well as application of best evidence supporting a modern caries management model.[8] This modern caries management model applies a preventive and conservative evidence-based approach, with a patient-centered risk-based disease management, focused on early detection of caries lesions and on the use of materials that promote remineralization and/or arresting of cavitated and noncavitated caries lesions.[9,10] Based on the lack of evidence regarding caries management in patients with SHCNs, and knowing that this group of patients, their conditions, and risk factors vary tremendously, personalized caries management is essential.

DISCUSSION
Caries Risk Assessment

Caries risk assessment is not only important for prevention of dental caries but also essential to guide the therapeutic approach, inform prognosis, and determine good strategies to better manage patients' oral health status. Assessing and reassessing patients' caries risk over time will help decide the management plan to stop the disease. Although risk-based prevention and disease management are now a recognized part of a modern caries management model,[11] enabling the clinician to develop a more cost-effective treatment,[9] data suggest a significant proportion of dentists are still not applying it in practice.[12] Part of this lack of adherence could be related to the fact that assessing level of risk involves subjective, expert-based, and not well-validated assessment tools to provide an accurate classification.[12]

Based on its importance, taking caries risk assessment into a context of patients with SHCNs is a good strategy to improve the success of their oral health management. Examples of its application in patients with SHCNs is found among children. Even though conditions are variable, in most existing risk forms, all children with SHCNs are considered in tandem. Examples of existing caries risk assessment tools that can be used include the ones by the American Association of Pediatric Dentistry (AAPD), American Dental Association (ADA), and Caries Management by Risk Assessment.[13–16] Caries risk questionnaires are easy to be answered and reflect on the patients' diet, oral hygiene habits, access to care, and dental and medical history. For young patients and patients with cognitive impairment, assessment should be conducted along with a family member, guardian, or caregiver and should include past and current caries experience, presence of plaque, frequency of consumption of carbohydrates, potential for a decrease in salivary flow rate, and exposure to protective factors, such as fluorides.[9,17] Risk factors will also vary and depend on the level and type of disability. For example, in children with autism spectrum disorders, these risk factors relate to diet, age, and especially to oral hygiene, and their behavior may be the major barrier to receiving dental care. Commonly, individuals with poor perceived behavior present higher odds of having unmet dental needs.[18] Medically

Table 1		
Caries risk factors associated with low-, moderate-, and high-caries-risk patients		
Caries Risk	**Low Caries Risk**	**Moderate to High Caries Risk**
Factors	No caries/no progression (3–5 y)	Current active caries lesions (current caries experience)
	Minimal past caries experience	Preexisting restorations (past caries experience)
	Low plaque accumulation	Placement of restorations since last visit
	Low frequency of sugar intake	High amount of plaque accumulation
	No salivary problems or reduction	Incremental frequency of carbohydrate consumption
	Adequate exposure to fluoride	Decrease in saliva flow
		Decrease in fluoride exposure

Data from Fontana M, Gonzalez-Cabezas C, Fitzgerald M. Cariology for the 21st century—current caries management concepts for dental practice. J Mich Dent Assoc 2013;April:32-40 and Fontana M. The clinical, environmental and behavioral factors that foster early childhood caries. Ped Dent 2015;37:217-25.

compromised and the vulnerable elderly and frail adult patients are also at increased risk for caries, often presenting multiple advanced lesions on root surfaces that need to be carefully assessed and addressed owing to their quick progression.[7,19]

Levels of caries risk are often divided into low, moderate, and high, with distinction between moderate and high caries risk often difficult and subjective to be determined. General factors associated with low-, and moderate- to high-caries-risk patients are listed in **Table 1**.

THERAPEUTIC OPTIONS: NONRESTORATIVE AND RESTORATIVE TREATMENTS FOR CARIES MANAGEMENT

Many modalities of nonrestorative and preventive measures can be offered to patients with SHCNs. Recent evidence-based clinical guidelines established by a panel of experts suggest nonrestorative treatments of caries lesions that are effective and can be used in conjunction or not with restorative treatment because of their effectiveness, safety, and feasibility.[20] In summary, the panel of experts lists the use of 38% silver diamine fluoride (SDF), sealants, 5% sodium fluoride varnish, 1.23% acidulated phosphate fluoride gel, and 5000 parts per million fluoride (ppm F) toothpaste or gel as the most effective interventions. In addition, the use of a 10% casein phosphopeptide amorphous calcium phosphate was not recommended. Here, these data are extrapolated from the general population to patients with SHCNs because of the absence of specific literature targeting these populations.

Fluoride and sealants are good examples of materials used for prevention and to improve success of caries management for the general population[2] and also in children and patients with SHCNs. Strong evidence shows that fluoride has topical ability to reduce dental caries' incidence, in both primary and permanent dentitions.[2,21] That includes fluoride products with clear effects on the primary and permanent dentition, as well as community water fluoridation.[22] Many strengths of fluoride toothpaste are available, but, typically, over-the-counter products are about 1000 ppm F, and higher concentrations are considered prescription-only medicine.[21] Largely used in school-based programs and at home, sodium fluoride rinses at 230 ppm F, for daily use, or at 900 ppm F, for weekly use, are another alternative to increase fluoride exposure and prevent caries lesions.[23] Importantly, fluoride management does not include only the type of product but also the establishment of its proper use. To achieve excellent mechanical plaque removal, toothbrushing using a manual or electric toothbrush with a fluoride toothpaste, for 2 minutes, twice daily is recommended. Knowing that fluoride's action is dose-dependent,[21] even over-the-counter toothpastes should have their rinse minimized to increase fluoride's protective effect. Additional challenges to the use of fluoride toothpastes may be imposed by sensory difficulties with flavor, texture, or taste sometimes presented by patients with autistic spectrum disorders.[18] Supervision is advised along with reinforcement of oral hygiene techniques to the caregivers and suggestion of more frequent recall visits.[3,18] Those recommendations present low-quality evidence and unclear benefits for patients with intellectual disabilities.[21] The choice of fluoride toothpaste concentration should be based on the patient's caries risk assessment, which also includes information about fluoride self-care exposure or professionally applied sources.[21] Risks of fluorosis and toxicity owing to ingestion of dentifrices should also be considered,[21] as well as risk of injuries during toothbrushing.[18] In general, because fluoride's effect is dose-dependent, higher concentration and increased exposure to fluoride are recommended for "at-home" and "in-office" uses when treating high-caries-risk patients. Examples of "at-home" regimens are the addition of fluoride rinses,[18,24] and/or high concentration fluoride toothpaste with the emphasis on avoiding the association of these 2 products to not dilute the prescription fluoride toothpaste concentration. Professionally applied fluoride products, such as gels and varnishes, every 3 to 6 months, are also excellent options to be added in the caries management plan for patients at moderate and especially at high caries risk.[25,26]

SDF has emerged as a promising therapeutic agent, in response to the need for materials that could modify the biofilm and enhance the remineralization process. This results in the arrest of cavitated coronal caries lesions and root surface lesions, while also being affordable, effective, safe, and easy to use[27] and being recommended for young children, vulnerable elderly and frail adults, and patients with SHCNs.[28] Although in the United States, SDF is only approved by the Food and Drug Administration as a professional desensitizer, systematic reviews[29,30] confirm its effectiveness as a caries-arresting agent in both primary and permanent dentition. Its in vivo mechanisms are still to be elucidated by ongoing studies, but the current evidence shows that SDF combines the remineralizing effects of fluoride[31] and the antibacterial effects of silver.[32] Importantly, in 2018, the AAPD developed an evidence-based recommendation regarding the application of 38% SDF to arrest cavitated caries lesions as part of the dental caries management strategies in children and adolescents, including those with SHCNs.[33] Application is simple and achieved under relative isolation, using a microbrush saturated by SDF solution to deliver the product to the cavitated surface (**Fig. 1**). Patients should avoid eating or drinking for 30 minutes after the application.[28] Reassessment is strongly recommended by examining the area of application after a few weeks or months. Arresting is noted when the cavitated area has hardened, and best results are achieved after reapplication, usually performed 6 months after the first intervention.[28] The biggest downside of SDF is the dark staining that occurs a few hours or days after its application; thus, it is not often recommended in esthetic areas[30] (**Fig. 2**). Despite the staining, without the need for caries removal, SDF represents an effective, affordable, and simple alternative for patients with SHCNs, presenting good parental acceptance when used in children.[34]

Dental sealants are proven to be one of the most efficient and cost-effective materials to prevent or control caries lesions,[2,35–37] being recommended over fluoride varnish to prevent caries lesions in occlusal surfaces, or to arrest noncavitated occlusal lesions.[35,38,39] They serve as a physical barrier on the tooth surface, preventing biofilm

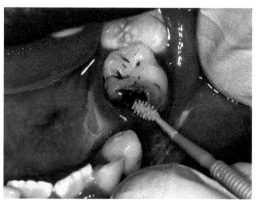

Fig. 1. SDF application on cavitated caries lesion. (*Courtesy of* Dr. C. Gonzalez and University of Michigan Global Initiatives in Oral and Craniofacial Health- Kenya program).

growth and reducing acidogenic bacterial nutrition.[40] Despite the strong evidence, cost-effectiveness, and large use in school-based programs,[36,37] its utilization remains low in dental clinics. Both resin-based and glass ionomer cement (GIC) sealants have been shown to prevent caries lesions.[41] GICs act by diffusing fluoride into the surrounding biofilms[42] and are hydrophilic, thus less technique sensitive in terms of isolation. When compared with resin-based sealants, GICs sealants are less resistant to attrition and present less retention to the surface, leading to higher need for replacement and monitoring.[38,39] Sealants can also be used to arrest microcavitated lesions but might need to be repaired yearly.[43] Along with resin infiltration and fluoride varnish, sealants are also recommended (after tooth separation) to be applied on noncavitated lesions in interproximal surfaces to arrest incipient approximal caries lesions in primary and permanent dentition.[20,44,45]

Another group of nonrestorative materials that have been applied to caries management is antimicrobials, mostly represented by chlorhexidine and polyols.[46] Regular use of xylitol or polyol combinations in chewing gum and lozenges can be an effective adjunct in coronal and root caries prevention,[2,47] because of the noncariogenic and antimicrobial properties of those chemical compounds. Overall, 0.12% chlorhexidine

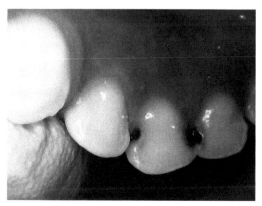

Fig. 2. Dark staining presented a few days after SDF application. (*Courtesy* of Dr. Margherita Fontana, DDS, PhD, Michigan.).

gluconate rinses present no effect on dental caries,[48] but professionally applied chlorhexidine/thymol varnishes are shown to be effective on the prevention and arresting of root caries lesions.[5,47] Comparatively, a recent systematic review has shown fluoride varnish, chlorhexidine varnish, and xylitol are less effective than SDF on root surfaces.[49] When discussing root caries, an important segment of patients with SHCNs is older individuals living in home care facilities. Because the majority of the evidence about fluoride comes from studies in children, several clinical trials have been conducted to generate data targeting independent living elderly individuals and those living in institutions.[50] Older individuals, generally, present high caries risk, especially to develop root caries,[51] because of a combination of exposed root surfaces, poor oral hygiene, frequent sugar intake, and use of medications reducing their salivary flow.[52] With insufficient evidence to recommend the use of any specific restorative material, such as amalgam, GIC, resin-modified glass ionomer cement (RMGIC), or composite resins for root caries,[53] and based on the high failure rates of root caries restorations, recent studies have focused on the use of fluoride.[54–57] Evidence shows that application of 5% sodium fluoride varnish, 3 to 4 times a year, is efficient to reduce caries in institutionalized older people,[54] especially when applied by a dental professional.[55] Recent data suggest biannual application of topical 38% SDF,[49,58] combined with oral health education, and use of 5000 ppm F toothpaste[59,60] is also effective to arrest root caries. In all of these strategies discussed thus far, the use of local anesthetic is unnecessary, and for those patients with challenges to cooperate for dental care in a routine setting, these conservative approaches are innovative.

When thinking about restorative treatments applied to caries management in special care dentistry, important consideration should be given to the decision-making process, rationale for the treatment, and management of the carious tissue. This is also going to include aspects related to behavior, access to care, level of disability (cognitive and/or motor), patient and family preferences and finances. Preservation of the tooth structure, its permanence in the mouth, and minimizing the cycle of re-restoration are desirable goals.[61] Restorative treatment should facilitate plaque control and management of caries at the affected surface, protect the pulp-dentine complex, and seal the area to promote lesion arresting, restore function, and promote esthetics.[61] When the cavitated carious lesions are noncleanable, minimally invasive restorative treatment should be used to reduce excessive tissue removal. If proper seal is achieved, bacterially contaminated or demineralized tissues close to the pulp do not need to be removed.[61] Texture and level of hardness should be used to guide caries removal instead of discoloration. Although distinction of level of hardness is difficult to achieve clinically, professionals should be trained to recognize different textures, ranging from soft, leathery, to firm and hard dentine, in order to proceed with a conservative approach.[5,61] Current evidence considers the need to reduce overtreatment and no longer advocates nonselective caries removal to hard dentin (also known as complete excavation or complete caries removal). The recommended approaches are based on the depth of the caries lesion and aim to protect the pulpal tissue. They are described as follows:

1. Selective removal to firm dentin (shallow lesions) in which the clinician uses a hand excavator to feel certain resistance and stops removing the tissue when reaches "leathery" dentine on the pulpal floor; the cavity margins are left hard (scratchy) after removal.
2. Selective removal to soft dentin (deep lesions) in which soft carious tissue is left over the pulp to avoid exposure, while peripheral enamel and dentine are prepared to hard dentine, to allow a tight seal and placement of a durable restoration.[61]

All these concepts of selective caries removal are in consonance with the minimal intervention dentistry philosophy that uses the atraumatic restorative treatment (ART) technique. The ART technique can be used in children, adults, and patients with SHCNs. It involves caries removal under local anesthesia, using only hand instruments, and restoring the cavity with high-viscosity adhesive materials, such as GIC or RMGIC. Higher success is achieved depending on the operator and on the number of surfaces. Dentists present higher success rates compared with students, and one-surface restorations show higher success rates.[62] Independent of the restorative material, current evidence strongly supports the use of a minimally invasive approach, aiming to delay the restorative cycle, preserving tooth structure, reducing the costs, and retaining teeth for a longer time.[61]

SUMMARY

Patients with SHCNs are composed of very diverse groups of individuals that are, in general, at an increased risk for dental caries. Because of the variety of health conditions and disabilities they might present, it is essential to assess their risk factors to determine an individualized plan of action to better manage caries in the short and long term. Ideally, minimally invasive dental procedures should be applied, with focus on prevention, caregivers' involvement, and patients' preferences. Attention to diet, with controlled sugar intake and frequency, and oral hygiene are also important measures to improve caries disease control and prevention. Nonrestorative materials that are low cost, efficient, and easy to apply are excellent options for patients with SHCNs, and clinicians should be aware of their use and supporting evidence. They include sealants and fluoride products, such as fluoride toothpaste (1000–1500 ppm F or 5000 ppm F), fluoride varnish, fluoride month rinses, chlorhexidine varnish, and more recently, SDF, that has emerged as a strongly evidence-based agent to arrest more advanced caries lesions. Recent and ongoing clinical trials and studies specially focused on caries management of root caries lesions in the elderly population are promising, adding new and important information to the management of this vulnerable population. Still, sparse evidence regarding caries risk management in patients with SHCNs is a barrier that needs to be overcome to generate more specific and consistent data to better serve these populations.

CLINICS CARE POINTS

- Caries risk assessment should be performed and reassessed over time in order to support a personalized caries management plan. For patients with special health care needs, an individualized plan considering the patient's preferences, frequent recalls, and close involvement of the caregivers is recommended.

- High-caries-risk patients should have increased fluoride exposure "in office" (eg, fluoride varnish every 3–6 months, sealants on occlusal surfaces), as well as an "at-home" regimen (eg, high-concentration fluoride toothpaste twice daily).

- Silver diamine fluoride, high-concentration fluoride toothpaste, fluoride varnish, and chlorhexidine varnish are examples of good nonrestorative alternatives to prevent and treat root caries.

- Silver diamine fluoride solution is a good nonrestorative alternative for cavitated coronal caries lesions and root surface lesions. Its application should be performed, biannually, under relative isolation and with the use of a microbrush. Reassessment to assure lesions are not progressing is highly recommended a few weeks or months after the intervention.

- When restorative treatments are necessary, selective caries removal using hand excavators is recommended. For shallow cavities, clinicians should remove tissue until reaching "leathery" dentine. In deep cavities, soft tissue can be left over the pulp to avoid damage. Good seal of the final restoration is essential to protect the tooth and assure success.

DISCLOSURE

The authors have nothing to disclose. Dr Fontana currently receives funding from the National Institutes of Health (NIH) in areas of caries risk assessment and caries management.

REFERENCES

1. Kassebaum NJ, Bernabe E, Dahiya M, et al. Global burden of untreated caries: a systematic review and meta regression. J Dent Res 2015;94:650–8.
2. Fontana M, Gonzalez-Cabezas C. Evidence-based dentistry caries risk assessment and disease management. Dent Clin North Am 2019;63:119–28.
3. Pini DM, Fröhlich PC, Rigo L. Oral health evaluation in special needs individuals. Einstein (Sao Paulo) 2016;14:501–7.
4. Khalid I, Chandrupatla SG, Kaye E, et al. Dental sealant prevalence among children with special health care needs: National Health and Nutrition Examination Survey (NHANES) 2013 to 2014. Pediatr Dent 2019;41:186–90.
5. Navarro Azevedo de Azeredo F, Silva Guimarães L, Azeredo A Antunes L, et al. Global prevalence of dental caries in athletes with intellectual disabilities: an epidemiological systematic review and meta-analysis. Spec Care Dentist 2019; 39:114–24.
6. Robertson MD, Schwendicke F, de Araujo MP, et al. Dental caries experience, care index and restorative index in children with learning disabilities and children without learning disabilities; a systematic review and meta-analysis. BMC Oral Health 2019;19:146.
7. Chávez EM, Wong LM, Subar P, et al. Dental care for geriatric and special needs populations. Dent Clin North Am 2018;62:245–67.
8. Fontana M, Eckert GJ, Keels MA, et al. Predicting caries in medical settings: risk factors in diverse infant groups. J Dent Res 2019;98:68–76.
9. Fontana M, Gonzalez-Cabezas C, Fitzgerald M. Cariology for the 21st century—current caries management concepts for dental practice. J Mich Dent Assoc 2013;April:32–40.
10. Evans RW, Clark P, Jia N. The caries management system: are preventive effects sustained postclinical trial? Community Dent Oral Epidemiol 2016;44:188–97.
11. Fontana M, Zero D. Assessing patients' caries risk. J Am Dent Assoc 2006;137: 1231–40.
12. Fontana M, Gonzalez-Cabezas C. Minimal intervention dentistry part 2. Caries risk assessment in adults. Br Dent J 2012;213:447–51.
13. American Academy of Pediatric Dentistry. Guideline on caries-risk assessment and management for infants, children, and adolescents. Pediatr Dent 2015;37: 132–9.
14. Ramos-Gomez FJ, Crall J, Gansky SA, et al. Caries risk assessment appropriate for the age 1 visit (infants and toddlers). J Calif Dent Assoc 2007;35:687–702.
15. Featherstone JD, Domejean-Orliaguet S, Jenson L, et al. Caries risk assessment in practice for age 6 through adult. J Calif Dent Assoc 2007;35:703-3.

16. Frank M, Keels MA, Quiñonez R, et al. Dental caries risk varies among subgroups of children with special health care needs. Pediatr Dent 2019;41:378–84.
17. Fontana M. The clinical, environmental and behavioral factors that foster early childhood caries. Pediatr Dent 2015;37:217–25.
18. Gandhi RP, Klein U. Autism spectrum disorders: an update on oral health management. J Evid Based Dent Pract 2014;14(Suppl):115–26.
19. Girestam Croonquist C, Dalum J, Skott P, et al. Effects of domiciliary professional oral care for care-dependent elderly in nursing homes – oral hygiene, gingival bleeding, root caries and nursing staff's oral health knowledge and attitudes. Clin Interv Aging 2020;15:1305–15.
20. Slayton RL, Urquhart O, Araujo MWB, et al. Evidence-based clinical practice guideline on nonrestorative treatments for carious lesions: a report from the American Dental Association. J Am Dent Assoc 2018;149:837–49.e9.
21. Walsh T, Worthington HV, Glenny AM, et al. Fluoride toothpastes of different concentrations for preventing dental caries. Cochrane Database Syst Rev 2019;3:CD007868.
22. Fontana M, Santiago E, Eckert GJ, et al. Risk factors of caries progression in a Hispanic school-age population. J Dent Res 2011;90:1189–96.
23. Marinho VC, Chong LY, Worthington HV, et al. Fluoride mouthrinses for preventing dental caries in children and adolescents. Cochrane Database Syst Rev 2016;7:CD002284.
24. Weyant RJ, Tracy SL, Anselmo TT, et al. Topical fluoride for caries prevention: executive summary of the updated clinical recommendations and supporting systematic review. J Am Dent Assoc 2013;144:1279–91.
25. Waldron C, Nunn J, Mac Giolla Phadraig C, et al. Oral hygiene interventions for people with intellectual disabilities. Cochrane Database Syst Rev 2019;5:CD012628.
26. Paris S, Banerjee A, Bottenberg P, et al. How to intervene in the caries process in older adults: a Joint ORCA and EFCD Expert Delphi Consensus Statement. Caries Res 2020;54:1–7.
27. Gao SS, Zhang S, Mei ML, et al. Caries remineralisation and arresting effect in children by professionally applied fluoride treatment—a systematic review. BMC Oral Health 2016;16:12.
28. Gao SS, Chen KJ, Duangthip D, et al. Arresting early childhood caries using silver and fluoride products – a randomized trial. J Dent 2020;103:103522.
29. Contreras V, Toro MJ, Elías-Boneta AR, et al. Effectiveness of silver diamine fluoride in caries prevention and arrest: a systematic literature review. Gen Dent 2017;65:22–9.
30. Crystal YO, Niederman R. Evidence-based dentistry update on silver diamine fluoride. Dent Clin North Am 2019;63:45–68.
31. Mei ML, Nudelman F, Marzec B, et al. Formation of fluorohydroxyapatite with silver diamine fluoride. J Dent Res 2017;96:1122–8.
32. Mei ML, Chu CH, Low KH, et al. Caries arresting effect of silver diamine fluoride on dentine carious lesion with S. mutans and L. acidophilus dual-species cariogenic biofilm. Med Oral Patol Oral Cir Bucal 2013;18:e824–31.
33. Use of silver diamine fluoride for dental caries management in children and adolescents, including those with special health care needs. Pediatr Dent 2018;40:152–61.
34. Almarwan M, Almawash A, AlBrekan A, et al. Parental acceptance for the use of silver diamine fluoride on their special health care-needs child's primary and permanent teeth. Clin Cosmet Investig Dent 2021;13:195–200.

35. Ahovuo-Saloranta A, Forss H, Hiiri A, et al. Pit and fissure sealants versus fluoride varnishes for preventing dental decay in the permanent teeth of children and adolescents. Cochrane Database Syst Rev 2016;2016:CD003067.
36. Gooch BF, Griffin SO, Gray SK, et al. Preventing dental caries through school-based sealant programs: updated recommendations and reviews of evidence. J Am Dent Assoc 2009;140:1356–65.
37. Griffin S, Naavaal S, Scherrer C, et al. School-based dental sealant programs prevent cavities and are cost-effective. Health Aff (Millwood) 2016;35:2233–40.
38. Oong EM, Griffin SO, Kohn WG, et al. The effect of dental sealants on bacteria levels in caries lesions. A review of the evidence. J Am Dent Assoc 2008;139: 271–8.
39. Wright JT, Tampi MP, Graham L, et al. Evidence-based clinical practice guideline for the use of pit-and-fissure sealants: a report of the American Dental Association and the American Academy of Pediatric Dentistry. J Am Dent Assoc 2016; 147:672–82.
40. Splieth CH, Christiansen J, Foster Page LA. Caries epidemiology and community dentistry: chances for future improvements in caries risk groups. Outcomes of the ORCA Saturday afternoon symposium, Greifswald, 2014. Part 1. Caries Res 2016;50:9–16.
41. Griffin SO, Oong E, Kohn W, et al. The effectiveness of sealants in managing caries lesions. J Dent Res 2008;87:169–74.
42. Mickenautsch S, Yengopal V. Caries-preventive effect of glass ionomer and resin-based fissure sealants on permanent teeth: an update of systematic review evidence. BMC Res Notes 2011;4.
43. Dorri M, Sunne SM, Walsh T, et al. Micro-invasive interventions for managing proximal dental decay in primary and permanent teeth. Cochrane Database Syst Rev 2015;(11):CD010431.
44. Wright JT, Tampi MP, Graham L, et al. Sealants for preventing and arresting pit-and-fissure occlusal caries in primary and permanent molars: a systematic review of randomized controlled trials—a report from the American Dental Association and the American Academy of Pediatric Dentistry. J Am Dent Assoc 2016;147: 631–45.
45. Meyer-Luckel H, Balbach A, Schikowsky C, et al. Pragmatic RCT on efficacy of proximal resin infiltration. J Dent Res 2016;95:531–6.
46. Schwendicke F, Jäger AM, Paris S, et al. Treating pit-and-fissure caries: a systematic review and network meta-analysis. J Dent Res 2015;94:522–33.
47. Walsh T, Oliveira-Neto JM, Moore D. Chlorhexidine treatment for the prevention of dental caries in children and adolescents. Cochrane Database Syst Rev 2015;4: CD008457.
48. Marsh PD. In sickness and in health—what does the oral microbiome mean to us? An ecological perspective. Adv Dent Res 2018;29:60–5.
49. Castelo R, Attik N, Catirse ABCEB, et al. Is there a preferable management for root caries in middle-aged and older adults? A systematic review. Br Dent J 2021. https://doi.org/10.1038/s41415-021-3003-2.
50. Patel R, Khan I, Pennington M, et al. Protocol for a randomised feasibility trial comparing fluoride interventions to prevent dental decay in older people in care homes (FInCH trial). BMC Oral Health 2021;21:302.
51. Griffin SO, Griffin PM, Swann JL, et al. New coronal caries in older adults: implications for prevention. J Dent Res 2005;84:715–20.
52. Steele JG, Sheiham A, Marcenes W, et al. Clinical and behavioural risk indicators for root caries in older people. Gerodontology 2001;18:95–101.

53. Hayes M, Brady P, Burke FM, et al. Failure rates of class V restorations in the man-agement of root caries in adults – a systematic review. Gerodontology 2016;33: 299–307.
54. Innes N, Evans D. Caries prevention for older people in residential care homes. Evid Based Dent 2009;10:83–7.
55. Tan HP, Lo ECM, Dyson JE, et al. A randomized trial on root caries prevention in elders. J Dent Res 2010;89:1086–90.
56. Li R, Lo ECM, Liu BY, et al. Randomized clinical trial on preventing root caries among community-dwelling elders. JDR Clin Trans Res 2017;2:66–72.
57. Zhang W, McGrath C, Lo ECM, et al. Silver diamine fluoride and education to pre-vent and arrest root caries among community-dwelling elders. Caries Res 2013; 47:284–90.
58. Grandjean ML, Maccarone NR, McKenna G, et al. Silver diamine fluoride (SDF) in the management of root caries in elders: a systematic review and meta-analysis. Swiss Dent J 2021;131:417–24.
59. León S, González K, Hugo FN, et al. High fluoride dentifrice for preventing and arresting root caries in community-dwelling older adults: a randomized controlled clinical trial. J Dent 2019;86:110–7.
60. Ekstrand KR, Poulsen JE, Hede B, et al. A randomized clinical trial of the anti-caries efficacy of 5,000 compared to 1,450 ppm fluoridated toothpaste on root caries lesions in elderly disabled nursing home residents. Caries Res 2013;47: 391–8.
61. Schwendicke F, Frencken JE, Bjørndal L, et al. Managing carious lesions: consensus recommendations on carious tissue removal. Adv Dent Res 2016; 28:58–67.
62. Jiang M, Fan Y, Li KY, et al. Factors affecting success rate of atraumatic restor-ative treatment (ART) restorations in children: a systematic review and meta-anal-ysis. J Dent 2021;104:103526.

The Impact of COVID-19 on the Oral Health of Patients with Special Needs

Ronald Ettinger, BDS, MDS, DDSc, DDSc(hc)[a],
Leonardo Marchini, DDS, MSD, PhD[b],*,
Samuel Zwetchkenbaum, DDS, MPH[c]

KEYWORDS

- Aged • Frail elderly • Special needs • Mental health • Oral health • COVID-19

KEY POINTS

- Among the populations most impacted by the COVID-19 pandemic were persons with special needs.
- Virtually all nonemergent dental care was strongly discouraged before the general population became eligible for receiving COVID-19 vaccinations.
- As a consequence of these new barriers, there was a large accumulation of dental needs in all populations, especially those with special needs, and particularly those requiring access to the operating room.
- The impact of COVID-19 resulted in dental offices being modified and upgraded to enhance infection control by adding a multitude of preventive equipment and procedures. Those procedures are sometimes overwhelming for persons with special needs.
- Alternatives to circumvent the impact of COVID-19 and reduce barriers to dental care for persons with special needs include teledentistry and noninvasive restorative techniques, as well as the use of silver diamine fluoride.

INTRODUCTION

The World Health Organization (WHO) on March 11, 2020 declared a global public health emergency because of infection by the severe acute respiratory syndrome coronavirus 2 (SARS-CoV-2), which causes COVID-19.[1] SARS-CoV-2 is a retrovirus

[a] Department of Prosthodontics, The University of Iowa College of Dentistry and Dental Clinics, N-409 Dental Science, Iowa City, IA 52242, USA; [b] Department of Preventive and Community Dentistry, The University of Iowa College of Dentistry and Dental Clinics, N337-1 Dental Science, Iowa City, IA 52242, USA; [c] Oral Health Program, Division of Community Health & Equity, Rhode Island Department of Health, Center for Preventive Services, 3 Capitol Hill, Suite 302, Providence, RI 02908, USA
* Corresponding author.
E-mail address: leonardo-marchini@uiowa.edu

with a single RNA strand presenting with 4 structural proteins: membrane protein, nucleocapsid protein, envelope small membrane protein, and spike glycoprotein.[2] The spike glycoprotein protrudes from the surface and binds to angiotensin converting enzyme 2 (ACE2) receptors to infect the epithelial cells of lung, heart, kidney, liver, gastrointestinal tract, and blood vessels. Under normal circumstances, ACE2 receptors help to regulate blood pressure, wound healing, and inflammation, as part of the renin-angiotensin-aldosterone system.[3] However, SARS-CoV-2 prevents ACE2 receptors from carrying out its normal function, which can cause severe inflammation and tissue injury.[4]

This virus is unique in that it has a high human-to-human transmission rate, but a lower fatality rate compared with other recent epidemics, such as the severe acute respiratory syndrome infection of 2003 and the Middle East respiratory syndrome infection of 2012. Although some persons infected by SARS-CoV-2 stay asymptomatic, COVID-19 symptoms include flulike symptoms, such as fever, dry cough, shortness of breath, headache, muscle pain, fatigue, anosmia, ageusia or dysgeusia, and diarrhea, which can progress to a severe form of viral pneumonia resulting in adult respiratory distress syndrome.[5] As SARS-CoV-2 spreads among different populations, it continually mutates into new variants. Several of these new variants have been shown to be more aggressively transmittable, as they spread more easily and quickly.[6] However, evidence has shown all the current vaccines are effective in preventing serious disease caused by these new variants.[7]

Although people of all ages may be infected, the majority (80%) of COVID-19 infections occur in adults aged 30 to 69, and mortality increases with age and the presence of comorbidities.[4] Death rates vary from 1 in 900 persons aged 18 to 29 years to 1 in 3 aged 85 years or older.[8] Most children and adolescents infected by SARS-CoV-2 have mild or no symptoms, but may have high viral loads and can spread the infection.[9] However, a small number can develop multisystem inflammatory syndrome.[10] The symptoms resemble Kawasaki disease, which is an acute febrile illness that has systemic vasculitis and involves the heart, resulting in coronary artery aneurysms leading to sudden death. Children presenting with these symptoms will need support in pediatric intensive care units to survive.[11]

Primary risk factors, besides older age, include hypertension, immunocompromised state, obesity, diabetes, chronic heart, liver, kidney and lung diseases, and also dementia.[12,13] According to the Centers for Disease Control and Prevention (CDC), persons with chronic medical conditions who are diagnosed with COVID-19 are 6 times more likely to need hospitalization, and 12 times more likely to die of the disease.[14] Persons with HIV infection or other immunocompromising conditions, such as those who have had a solid organ transplant, or who are taking immunosuppressant drugs owing to other conditions, are at very high risk of becoming infected by COVID-19, with a higher risk of dying of the disease, but they were not included in the large vaccine trials. However, recent data have shown many of these individuals do respond adequately to vaccinations for COVID-19, which may reduce their risk for infection if they receive the appropriate vaccinations.[15]

Before the development of vaccines, those most at risk were older adults living in long-term care facilities (LTCFs).[16] However, it must be noted persons with intellectual and developmental disabilities (IDD), especially those with Down syndrome and those who are immunocompromised or suffering from a major chronic disease, are at higher risk for COVID-19.[13] People with IDD and a positive diagnosis for COVID-19 showed higher rates of comorbidities, such as hypertension, heart disease, respiratory disease, and diabetes, which resulted in greater severity and mortality from COVID-19.[17] In fact, an analysis of claims data highlighted patients with developmental disorders of speech and language, developmental disorders of scholastic skills, and central auditory processing disorders had the highest odds of dying of COVID-19.[18]

Persons living in LTCFs are at higher risk for infection because of close communal living, as few residents have individual rooms, which does not allow appropriate social distancing.[13] Many of their caregivers have limited access to formal education and received minimal training, are required to use public transport, and live in multigenerational households that puts them at a higher risk of getting infected and transmitting the virus to the LTCFs residents.[19] Initially, there was a significant shortage of personal protective equipment (PPE) in LTCFs, which increased the risk of infection for the residents and staff.[16]

The initial impact of COVID-19 on society (March 2020) was to shut down businesses and quarantine populations, except for essential services. Hospitals and intensive care units were overrun by the first wave of severely sick patients with COVID-19, resulting in regional shortages of PPE and ventilators.[20] Business closures and quarantine caused job losses and consequently food insecurity[21] and loss of health insurance, including dental benefits.[22] More than 16 million persons lost their employer-sponsored dental insurance, which resulted in a decrease in routine checkups, hygiene visits, and fluoride applications, but an increase in tooth extractions.[23] Reduced incomes also forced many families to change to a cheaper and more cariogenic diet.[24] The isolation resulted in heightened stress levels, which increased tobacco, alcohol, and drug use.[25] There was also an unequal impact on different socioeconomic groups, for instance, white collar workers could use computers to work from home as opposed to many blue collar workers, who lost their jobs.[26] Many childcare facilities were closed and schools went virtual, which limited parents, especially women, from going to work. It was particularly stressful for children with learning disabilities and those with special needs, as well as their caregivers.[27]

Initially, all health care facilities, public and private, were encouraged to provide only emergency services, and elective procedures were suspended.[28] This situation had a significant impact on the provision of health care as well as oral health care.[29] The greatest impact was on the residents of LTCFs, where there were high rates of infection resulting in death.[16] The LTCFs responded by allowing only their salaried staff to enter the building and interact with the residents. Historically, persons living in LTCFs as well as those with special health care needs have received inadequate oral health care owing to a multitude of barriers, ranging from complex health histories to reduced socioeconomic status and transportation issues. The pandemic added another layer of barriers to providing appropriate dental care for these individuals.[30] The disruption of routine dental care and especially dental general anesthesia greatly impacted the population with special needs.[31]

The Special Care in Dentistry Association (SCDA) defines patients with special needs as those who have physical, medical, developmental, or cognitive conditions that limit their ability to receive routine dental care. This includes people of all ages. However, in this article, the authors focus only on adult patients, as children have different needs. The emphasis of this article is on the consequences of COVID-19 on oral health and disease among patients with special needs, as well as how dentists and dental care for this population have responded to the challenges posed by the pandemic.

CONSEQUENCES OF COVID-19 ON ORAL HEALTH AND DISEASE

At the beginning of the pandemic, as stated earlier, the CDC advised all elective medical procedures should be suspended in order to save limited supplies of PPE and allow all available health care personnel to focus on caring for the persons infected by COVID-19.[28] Dental offices were asked by the American Dental Association (ADA) and state health departments to limit care to emergency only and delay elective and routine care as the transmission mechanism of the virus was not fully understood.[29] However, this advice was based on literature showing medical procedures, such as intubation/extubation, bronchoscopy, ventilation, and airway suctioning, produced aerosols that transmitted infections.[32] In dentistry, most invasive procedures use ultrasonics, handpieces, air-water syringes, and lasers, which generate sprays, and a fraction of these sprays becomes aerosolized. By analogy with the medical procedures, the aerosols generated in dentistry were thought to be a potential mode of transmission of respiratory pathogens through saliva.[33,34] However, recent research has demonstrated SARS-CoV-2 transmission during dental treatments for asymptomatic patients is not as risky as initially thought, especially when infection-control procedures, such as high intraoral suction and preoperative rinses, are used.[35]

The suspension of elective dental care during the first 9 months of the pandemic delayed the provision of all routine care,[29,34] which allowed for an increase in the burden of dental and oral infections.[36] It has been reported the lockdown of the population was instrumental in causing food insecurity[21] and exacerbating depression, owing to job losses and isolation.[37] This scenario resulted in ingestion of a cheaper and more cariogenic diet,[24,38] which was associated with reduced self-care, including oral hygiene routines.[39] For persons with special needs who required help with their daily oral hygiene, another issue was that some caretakers were hesitant to help them with oral hygiene because of fear of infection.[30] Associated with reduced access to routine preventive dental services caused by the pandemic, the lack/reduction of oral hygiene routines may have led to further oral health deterioration among persons with special needs.[40]

Even among persons with special needs, some were at higher risk of oral health deterioration, for instance, persons with reduced manual dexterity, such as those persons who had rheumatoid arthritis, which makes it difficult for them to hold and manipulate a toothbrush. This also includes persons who have had a stroke that involved their dominant hand. Some of these individuals can perform their own oral hygiene procedures again by modifying toothbrushes to fit their particular problems. In some situations, using an electric toothbrush can help; others will need to depend on family and caregivers.[41] All of this population's problems were exacerbated by COVID-19, because of a lack of access to health care personnel and fear of infection by their caregivers.[30]

Individuals who have lost or are losing their vision may also be at risk for rapid oral health deterioration if they need help from others,[42] especially during the pandemic. Persons presenting with progressive cognitive decline, such as with Alzheimer disease and related dementias, as well as those with severe intellectual disabilities, who traditionally have required help with maintaining their activities of daily living (ADLs), including oral hygiene routines, became at greater risk for rapid oral health deterioration.[43] If they were living in communal housing, or LTCFs, they were at particular risk of being infected by COVID-19.[13] The reasons for this increased risk were these facilities did not have independent rooms for their residents to isolate those who were infected with COVID-19. Also, many of their caregivers lived in multigenerational houses, and many needed to use public transport, which put them at risk of being infected by COVID-19. These persons could not stop working for 2 weeks or more in order to abide by quarantine guidelines, and so carried the infection into the LTCFs.[19]

Persons who have cognitive impairment may have difficulties following CDC guidelines for safe practices during the COVID-19 pandemic. These individuals may not tolerate wearing masks, be unable to refrain from the need to physically touch surfaces, or understand appropriate social distancing, or the needs for using alcohol-based hand sanitizer or handwashing. This becomes a problem when these persons enter a dental office, and so require the staff and clinicians to be more vigilant and take extra precautions to protect themselves and other patients with appropriate countermeasures. However, the use of face masks and shields may stress people with cognitive impairment and create a barrier for hearing-impaired persons, because they cannot hear well or lip read, which may severely affect communication and informed consent.[19]

Another oral complication associated with the pandemic was an increase in the prevalence of sleep and awake bruxism.[44] During the pandemic, an electronic survey of a Brazilian adult population revealed bruxism increased significantly, and 47.8% of participants reported clenching and grinding caused them myofascial pain.[44] A possible cause for this increase in bruxism and oral facial pain was the stress caused by the pandemic lockdown, which was described as a major life stressor in another electronic survey.[45] In the same survey, COVID-19-related stress and depression were strongly correlated with orofacial pain.[45] During the pandemic in China, an online questionnaire, which included a general population, as well as patients with temporomandibular disorders (TMD), revealed persons with TMD reported higher levels of anxiety and depression than the general population.[46]

Several reports[47–49] have described various opportunistic fungal infections, recurrent and herpes simplex virus infection, unspecific oral ulcerations, and gingival infections associated with COVID-19. The most common explanation is that these oral infections are related to decreased salivary flow and an impaired immune system in patients with SARS-CoV-2 infection.[47] A recent article listed the most frequent oral manifestations presented by patients who have had COVID-19 infection. Overall, 84% of the patients had an oral manifestation, which were altered taste (42%), altered smell (39%), salivary gland ectasia (38%), white tongue (28%), dry mouth (24%), and facial muscle weakness (18%). Other oral manifestations were oral ulcers, abnormalities of the temporomandibular joint (TMJ), facial tingling, and trigeminal neuralgia.[49]

Access to operating room time for dental procedures, especially for children and adults with special needs, has been a problem long before the pandemic. However, because of COVID-19, hospitals limited access to their operating rooms even further, except for medical emergencies. Consequently, patients with special needs who could only be treated under sedation or general anesthesia had their appointments curtailed. When vaccines became available and hospitals began to allow elective procedures, competition from medical surgeons resuming elective medical procedures boosted long waiting times for oral health-related procedures, except for emergencies, such as significant pain, disseminated infection, and uncontrolled bleeding. Select health system requirements for pre-procedural COVID-19 testing also adversely impacted access to dental care for persons with special needs who could not tolerate such testing. The consequences of these delays have resulted in a higher rate of unrestorable teeth, which can only be extracted. It has been suggested COVID-19 has legitimized and sustained the bias for denial of access to operating rooms for dental procedures.[50]

HOW IS DENTISTRY ADAPTING TO PROVIDE CARE FOR PERSONS WITH SPECIAL NEEDS AS A RESULT OF THE PANDEMIC?

The initial response to the pandemic was to discontinue all routine and elective dental services, especially those of private practitioners.[29,34] As more knowledge about

SARS-CoV-2 became available, dental offices adapted by improving air filtration with HEPA (high-efficiency particulate air filters) aided with UV radiation.[51] Also, infection control procedures were enhanced by the use of nebulizers, upgraded PPE, which included face shields, eye-protection goggles, N95 respirators, impermeable gowns, and surgical caps[29] (**Fig. 1**). Protocols were developed, which included contacting the patient by telephone or interviewing the patient through virtual conferences to determine their health status and needs.[29] When dentists were allowed to open their offices for nonemergency care, patients were only allowed into the waiting room at the time of their appointment after a temperature check. Accompanying persons were discouraged, and all persons were required to wear masks and social distance from each other, unless they were related. Plexiglass shields were erected between the patients and the front desk staff (**Fig. 2**), who were also wearing masks. These new protocols were overwhelming, especially for older adults, and confusing for patients with special needs.[19] The face shields and N95 respirators reduced the ability of patients with limited hearing capacity to understand questions or directions from the clinician. However, for patients who were deaf or needed to lip read to understand verbal communications, the facial barriers simply precluded communication.[52]

A group of patients who have reacted negatively to the enhanced protections used by the dental profession during the pandemic are those with cognitive impairment, mental health issues, dementia, and developmental disabilities. These patients cannot process what is happening or why people are behaving so differently from what they were used to. Their reactions may have ranged from being afraid to being overtly aggressive and on occasion trying to look under the masks. As a result, it became more difficult to treat these persons in the ambulatory setting, as they became more dental phobic than previously.[19,52]

Patients with reduced mobility who were unable to use regular public transport also faced new barriers owing to COVID-19.[53] Wheelchair-adapted vehicles and ambulances were fully engaged in transporting patients with COVID-19 to and from

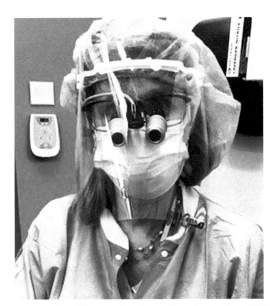

Fig. 1. Enhanced PPE used after COVID-19, included head covering, N95 mask covered by a surgical mask, and a face shield.

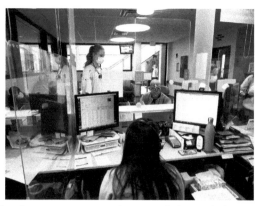

Fig. 2. Plexiglass barriers to protect patients and front desk personnel from cross-contamination by airborne particles.

hospitals, leaving no room for nonemergency transportations to and from dental facilities. If they were living in a LTCF, transportation supplied by the LTCF was only available to a hospital. Patients with reduced mobility often require more frequent recalls to maintain the health of their dentitions, and COVID-19 did not allow for these visits, increasing the patient's risk for rapid oral health deterioration.

When dental offices resumed routine care, in-office procedures were modified, which included the reduction of aerosol-generating procedures (AGPs), such as the use of handpieces and ultrasonic scalers. External suction devices (**Fig. 3**) were added to enhance aerosol reduction when combined with intraoral high-volume suction.[4] To reduce aerosols during professional tooth cleaning, hand scalers were used instead of ultrasonic scalers for plaque and calculus removal. To prevent aerosol production during caries removal, conservative procedures, such as the use of hand excavation, atraumatic restorative treatment (ART) technique, and silver diamine fluoride (SDF), were used to treat caries.[19]

The ART technique consists of manual soft caries excavation followed by the application of glass ionomer cement (**Fig. 4**) using cotton-roll isolation. ART is simple and might reduce patient anxiety and discomfort during caries removal. As a consequence, ART has been extremely successful for caries management for frail older adults and especially for persons with special needs. Long-term observations of ART-restored teeth showed similar survival rates to conventionally restored teeth.[54]

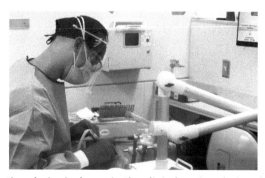

Fig. 3. External suction device is shown in the clinical setting during the restoration of a tooth, using a high-speed handpiece.

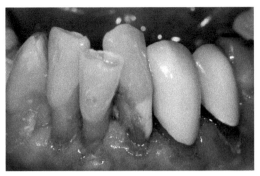

Fig. 4. A glass ionomer restoration done by the ART technique can be seen on tooth number 22 for a noncooperative, cognitively impaired 72-year-old patient showing poor plaque control, and chronic gingivitis with loss of attachment. ART was used to avoid generating aerosols by the use of a handpiece, as well as to provide a less traumatic experience for the patient, by reducing noise, and the use of local anesthetic.

When providing care outside of the dental office for frail older adults and persons with special needs or to patients with limited cooperation in the dental chair, ART has been shown to be particularly useful, cost-effective, and well accepted by patients.[55,56]

In many countries, SDF has been used to arrest and prevent caries for a long time, but it has only been available in the US market since 2014. SDF consists of 24% to 27% silver, 7.5% to 11.0% ammonia, and 5% to 6% fluoride.[57] Silver ions provide the antibacterial effect, by destroying the cell wall, denaturizing cytoplasmic enzymes, and inhibiting DNA replication. Fluoride and ammonia improve formation of fluorapatite and enhance remineralization.[58] Applying SDF is relatively easy and inexpensive, and it has been proven to be safe[59] (**Fig. 5**). As a result, SDF is very effective for caries prevention and arresting caries among frail older adults,[60,61] as well as for persons with special needs.[62]

Teledentistry was seldomly used before the pandemic. During the crisis, teledentistry was used to evaluate patients who were medically compromised and were unable

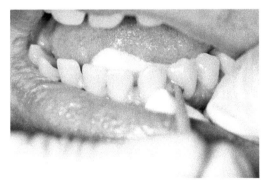

Fig. 5. The application of SDF for an intellectually disabled older adult with a history of interproximal caries. The lesion on tooth number 21 is situated partially subgingivally and will be very difficult to restore without crown lengthening, which was rejected by the power of attorney. The use of SDF will arrest the caries and allow for a less invasive procedure and so prolong the survival of the tooth.

to visit a dental office because of their health, increased risk for infection or because they were quarantined.[63] It also became an important tool for diagnosis, management, prevention, and provision of psychosocial support for patients through telephone and online consultation. For example, teledentistry is a cost-effective way to screen and evaluate any patient who has acute dental pain. These patients may need a prescription for analgesics, or if they have a facial swelling, an antibiotic. A decision needs to be made if the patient can be treated in the dental office or if he or she needs to be referred to a hospital emergency department that has a dental service. It also has become useful to monitor patients who have had an invasive procedure recently performed in the office. Teledentistry has also been used to guide patients and caregivers in self-management, especially for patients with bleeding disorders, such as hemophilia.[64] In addition, teledentistry can help to guide caregivers in placement of fluoride varnish and SDF for patients living in LTCFs.[65]

It has been suggested teledentistry is not a substitute for in-office treatment for the most common dental diseases. However, for patients living in rural areas, for patients living in LTCFs, and for those with mobility or transportation problems, teledentistry may be beneficial by providing oral health advice.[66] When using teledentistry, dentists should only consult with their own patients or with patients who have been referred to them. The protocol requires the dentist to properly identify the patient and have the patient's clinical record available. There is a need for the dentist to provide the patient with information about the limitations associated with a consultation via teledentistry. A detailed record of the appointment must be written into the patient's record at the end of the teledentistry appointment.[30]

The development of vaccines helped to change the environment. Persons living in LTCFs, those over the age of 80, persons with special needs, including persons with multiple comorbidities, and health care professionals were prioritized to receive the first available vaccinations. In most states, all hospital-based health professionals (including dentists) were vaccinated first. Community-based health professionals were the next to get vaccinated, and it included most of the dentists. However, in some states, dentists and other dental personnel were assessed at a lower tier among health care professionals to be vaccinated.[67] Concomitantly, more has been learned about the virus, and the guidelines from the CDC have been changed and updated. As a result, dental care has become normalized, but many of the procedures used for enhanced infection control have been incorporated into the "new normal." In addition, oral health professionals who care for patients with special needs are now needing to deal with the accumulated disease owing to nearly a year of limited care.[36]

The use of enhanced PPE and reduced scheduling owing to COVID-19 has resulted in increased baseline costs for dental practices. For these changes to be sustainable, patients and insurance companies will need to reimburse the dentist to cover these higher costs. Currently, some dental insurance companies are paying a limited fee to support teledentistry and providing some support for PPE acquisition. The ADA supports dentists charging a fee for the increased costs associated with treating patients during the pandemic. Oral health professionals and organized dentistry will need to lobby for changes in reimbursement rates from third-party companies to cover the additional costs.[68]

SUMMARY

Due to the spread of COVID-19, the WHO declared a global public health emergency (pandemic) in March 2020. Because of the pandemic, all non-urgent medical and dental care was suspended, and the shutdown disproportionally affected persons with special needs. The SCDA defines patients with special needs as those who have physical, medical, developmental, or cognitive conditions that limit their ability to receive routine dental care. This includes people of all ages. However, in this article, the authors focused only on adult patients.

Persons with special needs have a higher risk of morbidity and mortality if they became infected with COVID-19. The reasons for this are many of them have comorbidities and live in communal societies, where they receive supportive care from staff who themselves are at risk of infection because they live in multigenerational households and often need to use public transportation. Because of the pandemic, access to medical and dental services was limited to emergency care. Telehealth, including teledentistry, evolved as a method reaching these and other at-risk populations. Teledentistry was used to provide diagnosis, management, prevention, and provision of psychosocial support for these populations. Acute orofacial pain and/or infection could be managed by prescriptions of analgesics and antibiotics or, if necessary, referral to a hospital emergency department.

When elective dental care was resumed, dental offices adopted many procedures to minimize the risk of airborne infection. These procedures included improving the air filtration systems by using UV light and efficiency particulate air filters, more rigorous surface disinfection, enhanced PPE, including N-95 respirators, face shields, impermeable gowns, and head caps. Clinically, to reduce aerosol contamination, high-speed suction associated with extraoral suction devices was used. Also, more dentitions were hand scaled, and where possible, the concept of minimally invasive dentistry, including the ART technique and SDF, was used to manage caries.

CLINICS CARE POINTS

- The burden of oral health problems during the COVID-19 crisis was more intense for persons with special needs or residents of long-term care facilities.
- Changes in oral health care protocols owing to COVID-19, especially social distancing and having dental personnel wear face shields and masks, inhibited communication and exacerbated fears for persons with special needs (mainly those with hearing impairment, cognitive impairment and mental health problems).
- The expansion of the use of teledentistry was beneficial for the dentist as well as for persons with reduced access to dental facilities, especially those with special needs.
- The need to reduce aerosol-generating procedures resulted in the increased use of the atraumatic restorative treatment technique, the use of silver diamine fluoride, and the use of hand scalers for calculus and plaque removal.
- The enhanced preventive procedures and personal protective equipment, caused an increase in baseline costs for the dentist, which has made oral health care more expensive. Only some insurance companies have been prepared to subsidize these costs.

DISCLOSURE

The authors have nothing to disclose.

REFERENCES

1. Cucinotta D, Vanelli M. WHO declares COVID-19 a pandemic. Acta Biomed 2020;91(1):157–60.

2. Schoeman D, Fielding BC. Coronavirus envelope protein: current knowledge. Virol J 2019;16(1):69.
3. Hamming I, Timens W, Bulthuis ML, et al. Tissue distribution of ACE2 protein, the functional receptor for SARS coronavirus. A first step in understanding SARS pathogenesis. J Pathol 2004;203(2):631–7.
4. Lamberghini F, Testai FD. COVID-2019 fundamentals. J Am Dent Assoc 2021; 152(5):354–63.
5. Ng SL, Ong YS, Khaw KY, et al. Focused review: potential rare and atypical symptoms as indicator for targeted COVID-19 screening. Medicina (Kaunas) 2021;57(2). https://doi.org/10.3390/medicina57020189.
6. Center_for_Disease_Control_and_Prevention. About variants of the virus that causes COVID-19. 2021. Available at: https://www.cdc.gov/coronavirus/2019-ncov/transmission/variant.html. Accessed May 18, 2021.
7. Centers for Disease Control and P. What you should know about the possibility of COVID-19 illness after vaccination. 2021. Available at: https://www.cdc.gov/coronavirus/2019-ncov/vaccines/effectiveness/why-measure-effectiveness/breakthrough-cases.html. Accessed May 18, 3021.
8. Wiersinga WJ, Prescott HC. What is COVID-19? JAMA 2020;324(8):816.
9. Dong Y, Mo X, Hu Y, et al. Epidemiology of COVID-19 among children in China. Pediatrics 2020;145(6). https://doi.org/10.1542/peds.2020-0702.
10. Yonker LM, Neilan AM, Bartsch Y, et al. Pediatric severe acute respiratory syndrome coronavirus 2 (SARS-CoV-2): clinical presentation, infectivity, and immune responses. J Pediatr 2020;227:45–52.e5.
11. Keshavarz P, Yazdanpanah F, Azhdari S, et al. Coronavirus disease 2019 (COVID-19): a systematic review of 133 children presented with Kawasaki-like multisystem inflammatory syndrome. J Med Virol 2021. https://doi.org/10.1002/jmv.2706.
12. Killerby ME, Link-Gelles R, Haight SC, et al. Characteristics associated with hospitalization among patients with COVID-19-metropolitan Atlanta, Georgia, March-April 2020. MMWR Morb Mortal Wkly Rep 2020;69(25):790–4.
13. Center_for_Disease_Control_and_Prevention. People at increased risk. Updated April 20 2021. 2021. Available at: https://www.cdc.gov/coronavirus/2019-ncov/need-extra-precautions/index.html. Accessed May 18, 2021.
14. Stokes EK, Zambrano LD, Anderson KN, et al. Coronavirus disease 2019 case surveillance - United States, January 22-May 30, 2020. MMWR Morb Mortal Wkly Re 2020;69(24):759–65.
15. Geisen UM, Berner DK, Tran F, et al. Immunogenicity and safety of anti-SARS-CoV-2 mRNA vaccines in patients with chronic inflammatory conditions and immunosuppressive therapy in a monocentric cohort. Ann Rheum Dis 2021. https://doi.org/10.1136/annrheumdis-2021-220272. annrheumdis-2021–220272.
16. American Geriatrics Society (AGS) Policy Brief: COVID-19 and nursing homes. J Am Geriatr Soc 2020. https://doi.org/10.1111/jgs.16477.
17. Turk MA, Landes SD, Formica MK, et al. Intellectual and developmental disability and COVID-19 case-fatality trends: TriNetX analysis. Disabil Health J 2020;13(3): 100942.
18. FAIR_Health. Risk factors for COVID-19 mortality among privately insured patients: a claims data analysis. 2021. Available at: https://s3.amazonaws.com/media2.fairhealth.org/whitepaper/asset/Risk%20Factors%20for%20COVID-19%20Mortality%20among%20Privately%20Insured%20Patients%20-%20A%20Claims%20Data%20Analysis%20-%20A%20FAIR%20Health%20White%20Paper.pdf. Accessed June 29, 2021.

19. Marchini L, Ettinger RL. COVID-19 and geriatric dentistry: what will be the new-normal? Braz Dental Sci 2020;23(2):1–7.
20. Emanuel EJ, Persad G, Upshur R, et al. Fair allocation of scarce medical resources in the time of Covid-19. N Engl J Med 2020;382(21):2049–55.
21. Wolfson JA, Leung CW. Food insecurity and COVID-19: disparities in early effects for US adults. Nutrients 2020;12(6). https://doi.org/10.3390/nu12061648.
22. Levitt L. COVID-19 and massive job losses will test the US Health Insurance Safety Net. JAMA 2020;324(5):431–2.
23. Choi SE, Simon L, Riedy CA, et al. Modeling the impact of COVID-19 on dental insurance coverage and utilization. J Dent Res 2021;100(1):50–7.
24. Adams EL, Caccavale LJ, Smith D, et al. Food insecurity, the home food environment, and parent feeding practices in the era of COVID-19. Obesity (Silver Spring) 2020;28(11):2056–63.
25. DiClemente RJ, Capasso A, Ali SH, et al. Knowledge, beliefs, mental health, substance use, and behaviors related to the COVID-19 pandemic among US adults: a national online survey. Z Gesundh Wiss 2021;1–11. https://doi.org/10.1007/s10389-021-01564-4.
26. Lund S, Ellingrud K, Hancocks B, et al. Lives and livelihoods: assessing the near-term impact of COVID-19 on US workers. McKinsey Gloab Institute. Updated 2020. 2021. Available at: https://www.mckinsey.com/industries/public-and-social-sector/our-insights/lives-and-livelihoods-assessing-the-near-term-impact-of-covid-19-on-us-workers#. Accessed May 18, 2021.
27. Bellomo TR, Prasad S, Munzer T, et al. The impact of the COVID-19 pandemic on children with autism spectrum disorders. J Pediatr Rehabil Med 2020;13(3):349–54.
28. Zeegen EN, Yates AJ, Jevsevar DS. After the COVID-19 pandemic: returning to normalcy or returning to a new normal? J Arthroplasty 2020;35(7s):S37–41.
29. Ren YF, Rasubala L, Malmstrom H, et al. Dental care and oral health under the clouds of COVID-19. JDR Clin Trans Res 2020. https://doi.org/10.1177/2380084420924385. 2380084420924385.
30. Marchini L, Ettinger RL. Coronavirus disease 2019 and dental care for older adults: new barriers require unique solutions. J Am Dent Assoc 2020;151(12):881–4.
31. Okike I, Reid A, Woonsam K, et al. COVID-19 and the impact on child dental services in the UK. BMJ Paediatrics Open 2021;5(1):e000853.
32. Judson SD, Munster VJ. Nosocomial transmission of emerging viruses via aerosol-generating medical procedures. Viruses 2019;11(10). https://doi.org/10.3390/v11100940.
33. Kumar PS, Subramanian K. Demystifying the mist: sources of microbial bioload in dental aerosols. J Periodontol 2020;91(9):1113–22.
34. Marcenes W. The impact of the COVID-19 pandemic on dentistry. Community Dent Health 2020;37(4):239–41.
35. Meethil AP, Saraswat S, Chaudhary PP, et al. Sources of SARS-CoV-2 and other microorganisms in dental aerosols. J Dent Res 2021. https://doi.org/10.1177/00220345211015948. 220345211015948.
36. Baghizadeh Fini M. What dentists need to know about COVID-19. Oral Oncol 2020;105:104741.
37. Shah SMA, Mohammad D, Qureshi MFH, et al. Psychological responses and associated correlates of depression, anxiety and stress in a global population, during the coronavirus disease (COVID-19) pandemic. Community Ment Health J 2021;57(1):101–10.

38. Mattioli AV, Sciomer S, Cocchi C, et al. Quarantine during COVID-19 outbreak: changes in diet and physical activity increase the risk of cardiovascular disease. Nutr Metab Cardiovasc Dis 2020;30(9):1409–17.
39. Daly J, Black EAM. The impact of COVID-19 on population oral health. Community Dent Health 2020;37(4):236–8.
40. Limeres Posse J, van Harten MT, Mac Giolla Phadraig C, et al. The impact of the first wave of the COVID-19 pandemic on providing special care dentistry: a survey for dentists. Int J Environ Res Public Health 2021;18(6). https://doi.org/10.3390/ijerph18062970.
41. Treister N, Glick M. Rheumatoid arthritis: a review and suggested dental care considerations. J Am Dent Assoc 1999;130(5):689–98.
42. Schembri A, Fiske J. The implications of visual impairment in an elderly population in recognizing oral disease and maintaining oral health. Spec Care Dentist 2001;21(6):222–6.
43. Marchini L, Ettinger R, Hartshorn J. Personalized dental caries management for frail older adults and persons with special needs. Dent Clin North Am 2019; 63(4):631–51.
44. Pinzan-Vercelino CR, Freitas KM, Girão VM, et al. Does the use of face masks during the COVID-19 pandemic impact on oral hygiene habits, oral conditions, reasons to seek dental care and esthetic concerns? J Clin Exp Dentistry 2021;13(4): e369–75.
45. Saccomanno S, Bernabei M, Scoppa F, et al. Coronavirus lockdown as a major life stressor: does it affect TMD symptoms? Int J Environ Res Public Health 2020;17(23). https://doi.org/10.3390/ijerph17238907.
46. Wu Y, Xiong X, Fang X, et al. Psychological status of TMD patients, orthodontic patients and the general population during the COVID-19 pandemic. Psychol Health Med 2021;26(1):62–74.
47. Amorim Dos Santos J, Normando AGC, Carvalho da Silva RL, et al. Oral mucosal lesions in a COVID-19 patient: new signs or secondary manifestations? Int J Infect Dis 2020;97:326–8.
48. Egido-Moreno S, Valls-Roca-Umbert J, Jané-Salas E, et al. COVID-19 and oral lesions, short communication and review. J Clin Exp dentistry 2021;13(3):e287–94.
49. Gherlone EF, Polizzi E, Tetè G, et al. Frequent and persistent salivary gland ectasia and oral disease after COVID-19. J Dent Res 2021;100(5):464–71.
50. Vo AT, Casamassimo PS, Peng J, et al. Denial of operating room access for pediatric dental treatment: a national survey. Pediatr Dentistry 2021;43(1):33–41.
51. Zhao B, An N, Chen C. Using an air purifier as a supplementary protective measure in dental clinics during the coronavirus disease 2019 (COVID-19) pandemic. Infect Control Hosp Epidemiol 2021;42(4):493.
52. Marchini L, Ettinger RL. COVID-19 pandemics and oral health care for older adults. Spec Care Dentist 2020;40(3):329–31.
53. Cochran AL. Impacts of COVID-19 on access to transportation for people with disabilities. Transportation Res Interdiscip Perspect 2020;8:100263.
54. da Mata C, Allen PF, McKenna G, et al. Two-year survival of ART restorations placed in elderly patients: a randomised controlled clinical trial. J Dent 2015; 43(4):405–11.
55. da Mata C, Allen PF, Cronin M, et al. Cost-effectiveness of ART restorations in elderly adults: a randomized clinical trial. Community Dent Oral Epidemiol 2014;42(1):79–87.
56. da Mata C, Cronin M, O'Mahony D, et al. Subjective impact of minimally invasive dentistry in the oral health of older patients. Clin Oral Investig 2015;19(3):681–7.

57. Crystal YO, Niederman R. Evidence-based dentistry update on silver diamine fluoride. Dent Clin North Am 2019;63(1):45–68.
58. Peng JJ, Botelho MG, Matinlinna JP. Silver compounds used in dentistry for caries management: a review. J Dent 2012;40(7):531–41.
59. Horst JA, Ellenikiotis H, Milgrom PL. UCSF protocol for caries arrest using silver diamine fluoride: rationale, indications and consent. J Calif Dent Assoc 2016; 44(1):16–28.
60. Oliveira BH, Cunha-Cruz J, Rajendra A, et al. Controlling caries in exposed root surfaces with silver diamine fluoride: a systematic review with meta-analysis. J Am Dent Assoc 2018;149(8):671–9.e1.
61. Hendre AD, Taylor GW, Chavez EM, et al. A systematic review of silver diamine fluoride: effectiveness and application in older adults. Gerodontology 2017; 34(4):411–9.
62. Crystal YO, Marghalani AA, Ureles SD, et al. Use of silver diamine fluoride for dental caries management in children and adolescents, including those with special health care needs. Pediatr dentistry 2017;39(5):135–45.
63. Telles-Araujo GT, Caminha RDG, Kallás MS, et al. Teledentistry support in COVID-19 oral care. Clinics (Sao Paulo) 2020;75:e2030.
64. Pierce G, Dougall AA, Alkhayal Z, et al. WFH webinar: dental care for people with bleeding disorders during COVID-19 – what's changed? World Federation of Hemophilia. 2021. Available at: http://www1.wfh.org/publications/files/pdf-1773.pdf. Accessed June 29, 2021.
65. Versaci MB. COVID-19 pandemic shines light on telehealth services. New Dentist News 2020;24(3):1, 4.
66. Simon L. How will dentistry respond to the coronavirus disease 2019 (COVID-19) pandemic? JAMA Health Forum 2020;1(5):e200625.
67. Dooling K, McClung N, Chamberland M, et al. The Advisory Committee on Immunization Practices' Interim Recommendation for Allocating Initial Supplies of COVID-19 Vaccine - United States, 2020. MMWR Morb Mortal Wkly Re 2020; 69(49):1857–9.
68. American_Dental_Association. COVID-19 coding and billing interim guidance: PPE. American Dental Association. 2021. 2021. Available at: https://success. ada.org/~/media/CPS/Files/COVID/PPE_Coding_Billing_Guidance.pdf.   Accessed June 3, 2021.

Teledentistry for Patient-centered Screening and Assessment

Scott E.I. Howell, DMD, MPH[a],*, Brooke Fukuoka, DMD, FSCD[b]

KEYWORDS

- Disabilities • Elderly • Medically complex • Guided oral hygiene • Prevention
- Special health care needs • Teledentistry

KEY POINTS

- Providers can use teledentistry for patient populations that have historically faced barriers to accessing oral health services.
- Teledentistry allows oral health providers to work in coordinated teams that can communicate with one another using telecommunication technologies.
- Accurate data collection is important for a successful teledentistry visit and all members of the dental team should be trained on how to collect these data.
- Teledentistry can be used in a myriad of situations for any number of services, including guided oral hygiene, screenings, and examinations.
- Providers should be aware of the state laws and dental board policies to ensure they are using teledentistry within the law.

INTRODUCTION

People who have special health care needs (SHCN), such as those with complex medical conditions, the frail elderly, and people with disabilities, face myriad barriers when seeking dental care. Teledentistry is a more recent tool in our toolbox that allows us to take a more patient-centered approach and help our patients overcome these barriers. In any model that focuses on care for people with SHCN, adaptation is key. And the more tools we have in our toolbox, especially those that address patient needs, the more we can adapt our care delivery systems to ensure patients are getting the care they need and deserve. To help dental teams grow their adaptation

[a] A.T. Still University, Arizona School of Dentistry & Oral Health, 5835 E. Still Circle, Mesa, AZ 85206, USA; [b] Your Special Smiles PLLC, Family Health Services Idaho, 826 Eastland Drive, Twin Falls, ID 83338, USA
* Corresponding author.
E-mail address: showell@atsu.edu

Dent Clin N Am 66 (2022) 195–208
https://doi.org/10.1016/j.cden.2022.01.002
0011-8532/22/© 2022 Elsevier Inc. All rights reserved.

dental.theclinics.com

toolboxes, in the current article, we will discuss the barriers to care in this population and explore how teledentistry will help our patients overcome these barriers.

Nature of the Problem

By the year 2060, seniors will comprise 24% of the overall population.[1] 15% of adults aged 65 years and older are classified as frail, and the number of frail adults increases as age increases and the number of frail adults in long-term care was nearly double that of the general population.[2] This includes those who cannot care for themselves and have conditions that require around-the-clock care. Those living in long-term care facilities are often included as well. Individuals classified as medically complex are generally those who have multiple medical conditions, take numerous medications, or have numerous medical visits throughout the year, including multiple hospitalizations. Sixty percent of adults have 1 chronic disease, and 40% have 2 or more.[3] Acute conditions can lead to drastic decreases in quality of life and because these various medical conditions can be so volatile, patients often go without dental care.

We did not consider children in the current article because children generally have different systemic barriers to care. For example, pediatric dentists are trained to treat young people with disabilities, and state Medicaid programs offer comprehensive dental coverage for children. For adults with disabilities, dental training is less ubiquitous, and state Medicaid programs may or may not cover dental care. Approximately 1 in 4 adults have disabilities,[4] and the level of disability varies. When considering dental care in this population, those with more severe disabilities typically have greater levels of oral disease.

Rates of dental disease for people with SHCN are staggering. Ninety-three percent of seniors have experienced caries, and 18% have untreated caries.[5] In patients with complex medical conditions, we often see higher rates of xerostomia because of polypharmacy or certain medical treatments (eg, radiation for head and neck cancer). In one review, 37% of adults aged 60 years and older were taking 5 or more prescription medications.[6] Although individuals with head and neck cancer are more likely to live longer than 40 years ago, rates of head and neck cancer have increased since 2000.[7] As such, we see more people with a history of head and neck radiation in dental clinics, and they are also highly susceptible to radiation caries. For people with disabilities, periodontal disease approaches 70%, and caries rates are as high as 95%.[8] Because individuals with disabilities are living longer, dental disease rates will continue to increase.[9]

These populations not only face increased risk factors but they also have unique barriers to care. Even if all were welcomed into brick-and-mortar clinics, barriers exist. Unfortunately for health care, if you build it, they don't always come. There may be myriad reasons why people lack access to those clinics. One such reason is a lack of adequate funding. For many patients in this population, their only dental coverage is Medicaid. According to the American Dental Association (ADA), the percentage of dentists who take Medicaid varies from state to state. For example, less than 16% of dentists take Medicaid in New Hampshire, but more than 77% do so in Iowa.[10] When considered by specialty, the most common Medicaid providers are pediatric dentists, and adult patients with SHCN are not usually treated by pediatric dentists. Although nearly three-quarters of seniors indicate they will visit the dentist in the next year, less than half actually do.[11] Cost is the most common reported reason for not going to the dentist, but inconvenient locations/times or trouble finding a dentist account for 9% and 11%, respectively, of reasons for not going to the dentist.[11]

Issues with going to the dentist are compounded for patients with SHCN because they may be unable to drive, have a caregiver who works elsewhere during normal dental hours or are unable to communicate their needs because of their disability. Therefore, teledentistry can have a unique and crucial role for patients with SHCN. So let us dive into what teledentistry is and how it can be used to address the oral health needs of this population.

Basics and History of Teledentistry

Teledentistry can be defined as using technology to connect oral health providers in one location to patients in different locations. These oral health providers can be dentists, hygienists, assistants, or dental therapists. Further, teledentistry is not a procedure; instead, it is a term used to describe the way that we communicate. It usually involves electronic health records, an Internet connection, telecommunications technology, and digital images. As several resources already describe the basic definitions and concepts of teledentistry in great detail,[12,13] we have not included this information in the current article.

However, readers should be aware that there are 4 primary teledentistry modalities: synchronous, asynchronous, remote patient monitoring, and mobile health. A variety of clinical models exist using one (or more) of these modalities. Historically, most teledentistry models used a third person who was with the patients collecting appropriate medical and dental records. That person then communicated with the dentist about clinical findings. These third parties could be dental or medical providers, such as dental hygienists or nurses. The COVID-19 pandemic provided an impetus for oral health providers to communicate directly with their patients through video conferencing without having that third person in physical proximity to patients to collect clinical records.

Although the pandemic put a spotlight on teledentistry, the concept is not new. Teledentistry has mostly been used in the community and public health sectors. In the first reported teledentistry project, the US military used it to decrease travel times and increase the quality of care.[14] In the early 2010s, Dr. Paul Glassman and his colleagues at the University of the Pacific introduced the virtual dental home.[15] These early uses of teledentistry within the community and public health have created strong foundations for teledentistry in the private sector.

Although the focus of the current article is on the patient-centered approach affected by teledentistry, there are also benefits to dental clinics. Teledentistry allows everyone on the dental team to work at the top of their scope, and it allows clinics to maximize revenue. Dentists train for several years to evaluate patients and to treat the signs and symptoms of disease. Teledentistry allows clinics to shift how dentists spend their time. When dental chairs are filled with patients who need examinations or preventive care, clinic revenue is limited. Dental chairs, ideally, should be filled with patients who need physical intervention or evaluation. When procedures that generate lower revenue are moved out of the clinic and into the community, revenue can increase. For example, when hygienists are with patients collecting clinical records, they can also provide any necessary preventive or periodontal therapy and spend time reviewing important information related to oral hygiene. As these procedures generate much less revenue than procedures performed by dentists, keeping them in the dental clinic limits its revenue. For these reasons, teledentistry is financially beneficial for the dental clinic.

DISCUSSION
Necessary Information for a Teledentistry Visit

The authors of the current article have a combined experience of nearly a decade of teledentistry use in our practices, and most of those experiences involved a third party who was with the patient. However, we anticipate direct-to-patient encounters, whereby oral health professionals and patients meet through video conference, will become more common. Direct-to-patient visits work well for treatment plan presentations, postoperative evaluations, and other types of visits that may not require a hands-on approach. For patients with disabilities who have anxiety about going to dental clinics, direct-to-patient visits can be a useful approach to introduce patients to the dental clinic. Patients can meet the dentist and other staff and virtually tour the clinic so that when they physically go to the clinic there will be fewer unknowns, which would otherwise increase their anxiety.

As the third-party model is more commonly used, our focus will shift to preparing for this type of model. When describing its policy on teledentistry, the ADA states, "The ADA believes that examinations performed using teledentistry can be an effective way to extend the reach of dental professionals."[12] They also specify that "services delivered via teledentistry must be consistent with how they would be delivered in-person."[12] Given that dentistry is very hands-on in nature, many may find it difficult to understand how virtual examinations can be consistent with in-person examinations. One of the most important aspects of a virtual visit is the camera, including an intraoral camera, an extraoral camera, and a webcam. There are numerous cameras on the market and it is not necessary to spend thousands of dollars to get quality images. Importantly, when using teledentistry to evaluate patients from a distance, the data being collected should be consistent with in-person examinations as suggested by the ADA. Unfortunately, it is difficult to highlight every nuance of a teledentistry visit because state laws vary tremendously in terms of what is allowable and necessary. However, we do have some recommendations.

First, whoever is collecting data on the other end of the camera from the dentist should be someone the dentist trusts. This other individual should also be calibrated to what the dentist would do if actually there in person. For instance, if the dentist asks specific questions of every new patient, then the other individual should be asking those same questions. If the dentist wants to view certain parts of the mouth, then the third party should know how to capture images of those parts of the mouth with the intraoral camera. Clinical photos or videos should have several key qualities. Specifically, the teeth must be as dry as possible, and images of all necessary anatomic landmarks must be captured. If these landmarks cannot be captured in a single image, multiple images should be obtained. A minimum of 3 photos—buccal/facial, incisal/occlusal, and lingual/palatal—should be captured for any tooth in question. Soft tissue that is associated with any tooth in question should also be captured. When present, we also recommend capturing the mucogingival junction. See **Fig. 1**.

If the third party is recording videos, it is important that videos be recorded smoothly and slowly. We also recommend recording the entire mouth in a series of videos rather than in a single video to reduce saliva accumulation and patient exhaustion. The longer

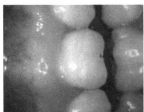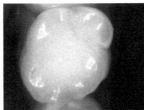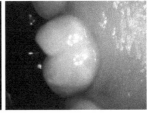

Fig. 1. A series of 3 images of tooth #3. These images capture all the necessary hard tissue and soft tissue needed to accurately assess and diagnose this tooth.

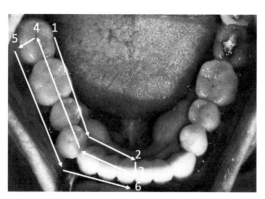

Fig. 2. The recommended s-shape when recording a video of the mouth. Start at the distal lingual of the most posterior tooth (1) then move to the midline (2), rotate to the incisal edge (3), move the camera posteriorly to the most distal tooth (4), rotate to the buccal and have the patient bite halfway down while using the camera to retract the cheek (5), and then move the camera to the midline on the facial (6).

the camera is in the mouth the more the patient is going to salivate, which will ultimately obscure what the provider needs to see. As the patient gets tired because the mouth is staying open, they may close their mouth on the camera, making it difficult to see the necessary anatomic landmarks. One method is to use an s-shaped figure that starts at the most distal lingual aspect of the. See **Fig. 2**.

Based on the patient's chief complaint, the third party may collect additional information, such as probing depths, vitality testing with Endo Ice, or tooth mobility. Depending on the scope of practice and the state's dental practice act, these various objective findings are often be collected by hygienists; however, the final diagnosis (usually) rests with the dentist.

As previously mentioned, it is very important that dentists and third parties are calibrated. If third parties do not collect accurate or enough information for dentists to form a diagnosis, dentists may be unable to finish and bill for the examination. Regardless of whether the examination was conducted in-person or through teledentistry, it may be viewed as unethical, or possibly illegal, to bill patients or their insurance for examinations lacking enough data to make a diagnosis. Therefore, checklists should be used to ensure that third parties collect all the necessary information. For example, the checklist could include questions the third party should ask patients about their chief complaint to help identify the appropriate clinical data that needs to be collected. In situations whereby third parties connect with dentists synchronously, the dentists can direct third parties to collect specific records. In asynchronous situations, whereby dentists review records later, checklists are especially important because the third party may no longer be with the patient when the dentist reviews the records. See **Box 1**.

Therefore, an important aspect of record collection is record collection training, which may include proper use of intraoral cameras or how to accurately conduct vitality tests on teeth using Endo Ice. A major mistake dentists can make is sending third parties into the field with no training on how to use intraoral cameras. To obtain correct intraoral images, the setup of the patient in relation to the computer is important because the third party must be able to easily see the computer while moving the camera around in the patient's mouth. Ideally, the computer will be in the direct line of sight of the third party, typically behind the patient's head. Another important factor of

---

Box 1
Dental pain and/or abscess checklist

1. Is there pain? Swelling? Both?
2. How severe is the pain/swelling?
   a. Is it limited to just around the gums? Can you visualize and/or palpate it extraorally?
3. How large is the swelling?
4. Is the swelling indurated or fluctuant?
5. Is there any purulence?
6. When did pain/swelling begin?
7. Is the pain spontaneous, wake the patient up or at night, or does it only occur when eating/drinking?
8. Has the pain/swelling changed?

   a. If the pain/swelling has changed, what time frame did it occur in?
9. Is the patient having any difficulty talking, breathing, swallowing, or opening?
10. Are there any other structures affected?
    a. Maxillary: Is the tissue around the eye affected?
    b. Mandibular: Can you palpate the inferior border of the mandible?
    c. Intraoral: Is the uvula dropping to the tongue? Is the uvula deviating? Is the tongue being elevated?
11. Is there any lymphadenopathy? Is there a fever? Does the patient seem toxic?
12. Have any images or laboratories been completed?
13. What is the white blood cell count, if known?
14. If the patient is unable to communicate is their behavior different than normal? Are they really grumpy, want to be left alone, not behaving like they usually do, etc?

---

record collection is that all images should be obtained using a secure fulcrum. Usually, when providers press the capture button on the camera, that action causes the camera to move. Without a secure fulcrum, which often uses the provider's nondominant hand, the image will be blurry, or the camera will move in such a way that does not capture the necessary anatomic landmarks. Lastly, to get consistent photos, the camera should always be at a similar angle to the arch or tooth being photographed. See **Fig. 3** and **4**. By following these simple steps, the teledentistry visit will be more productive and efficient.

Examples of Teledentistry in Practice

Now, we would like to provide an example of how we personally use teledentistry. In Dr. Fukuoka's practice, Your Special Smiles PLLC, teledentistry is used for a variety of purposes. The most common uses are for guided oral hygiene (GOH), screenings, periodic examinations, and limited examinations.

Guided Oral Hygiene

The concept of GOH was defined by a collaborative group consisting of members from Your Special Smiles PLLC (YSS), Idaho State University Dental Hygiene Sciences, the Idaho Oral Health Program, and Paul Glassman as the following:

GOH utilizes audio and video technology to guide a patient or caregiver as they carry out self-care oral hygiene on a regularly scheduled basis. GOH is patient-

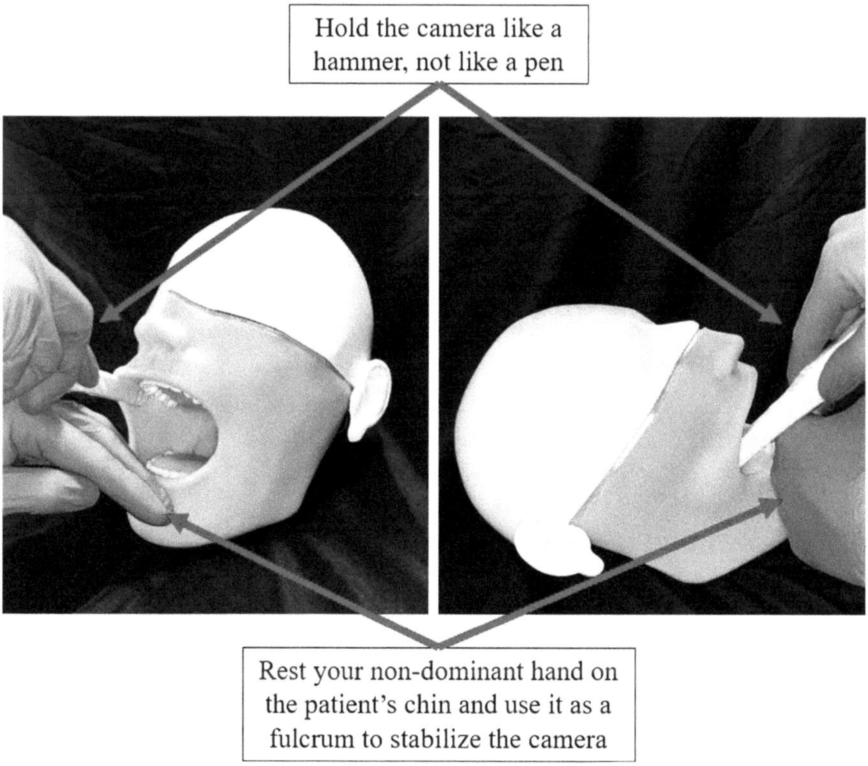

Hold the camera like a hammer, not like a pen

Rest your non-dominant hand on the patient's chin and use it as a fulcrum to stabilize the camera

Fig. 3. In these images, the provider is using the nondominant hand to provide a secure fulcrum so that the camera remains steady.

specific and does not apply to the use of generic prerecorded oral hygiene instruction videos. GOH is a specific service and may be delivered separately or as part of a remote oral health support program. GOH can be represented by a combination of oral hygiene instructions (D1330) and synchronous teledentistry (D9995).

Although GOH can be a one-on-one service provided directly to patients, it is currently used to train caregivers who assist patients with their homecare. This personalized guidance enables caregivers to carry out customized hygiene plans, learn various homecare techniques, and gain confidence in providing oral hygiene for dependent adults. In addition to being a training tool, GOH is also an awareness service. Regular sessions keep oral hygiene at the forefront of the mind of caregivers and patients. At YSS, we schedule GOH every 2 months for each patient, and each session lasts between 20 minutes and 1 hour.

A GOH program begins with the dentist reviewing the patient's medical history followed by appropriate consultations and visits with the patient if needed. The dentist then writes out any needed modifications. Next, clinical data are gathered, and the dentist or hygienist develops a customized hygiene plan and instrument list. From there, the hygienist or a specifically trained assistant can use synchronous teledentistry to help the caregivers carry out the customized hygiene plan. The hygienist or dentist can monitor this plan and the patient's oral health by periodically joining the synchronous sessions or by using asynchronous teledentistry to view recorded sessions later. See **Fig. 5**.

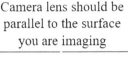

Camera lens should be parallel to the surface you are imaging

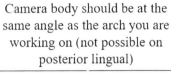

Camera body should be at the same angle as the arch you are working on (not possible on posterior lingual)

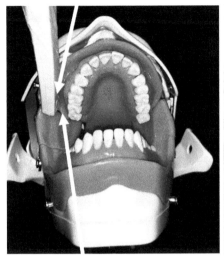

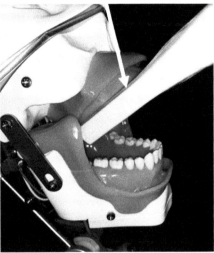

Camera should be about 1 inch away from the surface you are imaging

Fig. 4. In these images, the provider is holding the camera in a way that limits the distortion of the photo so that an accurate assessment and diagnosis can be made.

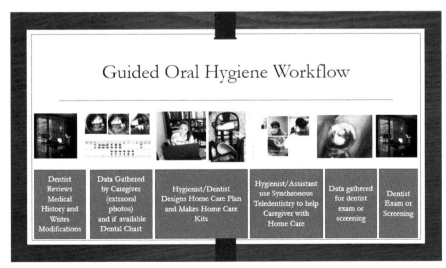

Fig. 5. This image illustrates the workflow that YSS uses when providing GOH services.

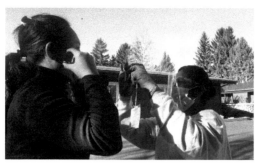

Fig. 6. *A hygienist training a caregiver in person on extraoral photography in the facility parking lot during the COVID-19 pandemic.*

Videos are an important aspect of GOH. Extraoral videos allow providers to see the patient's reactions. Intraoral videos help caregivers, patients, and providers find areas that were missed. Generally, intraoral videos are obtained one quadrant at a time, and the person taking the video verbalizes whereby the camera is recording. For example, the person may say, "We are now on the buccal of the upper right." This verbalization orients the provider when viewing the videos. When necessary, these videos can also be used for other modalities, such as screenings or examinations. Caregiver training is an important aspect of making GOH successful. Laminated training sheets that can be cleaned and reused have basic dental terminology and are provided as cheat sheets during the delivery of GOH services. A YSS hygienist also meets with caregivers in person and trains them on infection control, intraoral and extraoral photography, and proper use of the technology. See **Fig. 6**.

The following technologies are used at YSS: the Lester Dine (Dine Corp., Palm Beach Gardens, FL) extraoral camera for full mouth still shots, the MouthWatch intraoral camera (Metuchen, NJ) for intraoral photos and videos, TeleDent by MouthWatch as the teledentistry platform, a Surface Pro 4 tablet with Windows 10 Pro (Microsoft, Redmond, WA), and a Verizon MiFi 5G hotspot (New York, NY).

We have also found the following products useful for GOH sessions. Just Right 5000 ppm fluoride gel (Elevate Oral Care, West Palm Beach, FL) is dosed so the caregiver gets consistent amounts of gel with every pump. MI Paste from GC America (Chicago, IL) has multiple flavor options and provides calcium and phosphate for those who have decreased saliva. Bite blocks from Medline (Northfield, IL) or the Specialized Care Company (Hampton, NH) are used to help the patient keep the mouth open while the caregiver provides oral hygiene. Three-sided manual toothbrushes, such as the Surround Toothbrush (Specialized Care Co.), the Collis Curve (Brownsville, TX), and the DenTrust (Toledo, OR), can be used for patients who have limited cooperation. We also like the Triple Bristle (Dayton, TN) is a 3-sided electric toothbrush that is easy to use and clean. For those with sensitive or friable gingiva, TePe Special Care (Anaheim, CA) ultrasoft toothbrushes work well. It is also valuable to have various interproximal cleaners available. A cordless Waterpik (Waterpik, Inc., Fort Collins, CO) and an emesis basin are helpful to clean teeth while patients remain in a chair, and adult bibs are used to keep the patient's clothes clean. Storage of these instruments is also important. All instruments are cleaned before storage, are stored whereby they can dry, and are kept separate from the instruments of other residents when sharing a room or bathroom. Keeping track of oral hygiene products is easier when each resident have their own travel case. See **Fig. 7**.

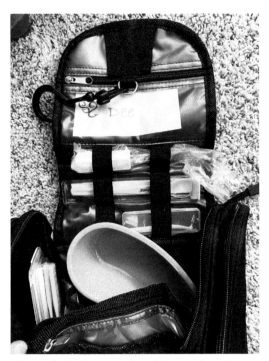

Fig. 7. An example of an individual oral hygiene kit that allows for organization, labeling, and air drying.

The key factor for successful GOH is the connection between the caregiver and the oral health provider. There are various ways to cultivate this connection. Training improves caregiver comfort and provides regular reminders about the importance of oral hygiene. Providers who are thinking about offering GOH should investigate multiple options and program designs to find what will work best for the patients, the providers, and the practice. For additional information about GOH, please visit the YSS website: https://www.yourspecialsmiles.com/short-clips-and-tips.

Screenings and Examinations

For some patients with SHCN, being at home in a comfortable environment results in increased cooperation, which in turn decreases the need for sedation or protective stabilization. When combined with allied health professionals willing to provide community-based treatment, the use of teledentistry can improve access to preventive care for patients who struggle with in-person visits. For the providers at YSS, the dentist must screen the patient for potential medical complications before providing any services. This screening involves live synchronous interactions between the dentist and the patient and a thorough review of the medical history. After the dentist has screened for potential complications, the hygienist can then provide preventive services before finishing collecting data to complete the comprehensive examination. See **Fig. 8** and **9**.

When examinations are conducted through teledentistry and videos of the patient's mouth have been recorded, providers can "pause" the videos to look at teeth for as long as needed. This ability is especially helpful for patients who do not hold still, making in-person examination difficult. Teledentistry is not used for every patient, every

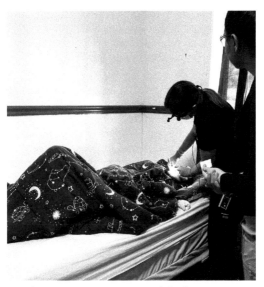

Fig. 8. A hygienist provides preventative services while the patient remains in his bed. This patient was able to receive regular hygiene services without sedation or stabilization by meeting him in a place he is comfortable.

time. Instead, YSS uses a hybrid approach, sometimes conducting examinations in person and sometimes through teledentistry. The approach used is based on patient needs, provider availability, and what was successful in previous examinations. There are also times when an examination starts with teledentistry but ends with an in-person visit. Having this flexibility to shift between approaches has been beneficial for providers and patients.

Even with limited examinations, teledentistry has increased efficiency. Before providers see patients in person, they can review medical history, send appropriate consultations, diagnose (or at least form a clinical impression for the problem), and generate treatment plans. With that information, providers can determine the appropriate location for additional examination or treatment of patients. This use of teledentistry saves time, especially when patients are ultimately referred to specialists.

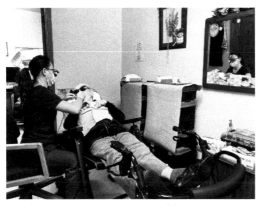

Fig. 9. A hygienist provides dental services in a portable clinic eliminating the need for the stressful drive to the dental office.

Teledentistry also allows providers to talk with patient guardians and primary care providers before seeing the patient in person, eliminating the need to contact multiple parties when the patient is in the dental chair or, worse, having to schedule subsequent in-person visits due to inability to obtain consent.

Challenges and Recommendations

Because teledentistry is still a relatively new approach for delivering care, state legislatures or dental boards may be hesitant to modify dental practice acts to permit the use of teledentistry. Therefore, when considering whether to incorporate teledentistry into clinical practice, providers should review their practice acts and check with their state boards to ensure they are practicing within the law. Providers should also check with their state Medicaid or private insurance programs to confirm which procedures are reimbursed when using teledentistry. Finally, providers should check with their malpractice carriers because some may not cover care provided through teledentistry.

In terms of state laws, some states have enacted legislation that makes the teledentistry process very prescriptive, which may limit the provider's capacity to connect with patients. Therefore, we encourage state legislatures and state dental boards to avoid developing teledentistry rules and regulations that make using teledentistry burdensome. It is important to remember that an in-person examination and an examination conducted through teledentistry have the same goal—to determine the diagnosis and develop a plan. We are simply using different tools to reach this goal.

Another challenge associated with teledentistry is how data are collected. Sometimes, due to the hands-on nature of dentistry, it is difficult for dentists to trust nondentists in data collection. What is important to remember is that the quality of the data is more important than who collects the data. With in-person models, dentists often work with hygienists and assistants to collect data as a team. For example, before a dentist physically examines a patient, a team member may chart existing restorations. It is also common for a hygienist to identify suspect pathology, who then alerts the dentist before the examination. Teledentistry simply takes this model, uses technology, and spreads it over a distance. We suggest that dental education can play a role to help overcome this challenge. Dental schools should be educating future dentists on how to diagnose using digital records. Allied dental health programs (eg, dental hygiene) should educate their students in quality digital data collection in conjunction with the physical data collection that already occurs. All dental education should teach their students how to work in collaborative and teledentistry-based models.

Lastly, providers may feel that if an examination was initiated using teledentistry then it must be completed with only the information provided. This is not true. A provider can request more information be gathered. Alternatively, it is entirely possible for a provider to physically examine a patient in conjunction with teledentistry. Some might argue that this defeats the purpose of teledentistry, but we have found tremendous value in these services within our respective communities as the teledentistry visit lays the foundation for a more efficient in-person visit. We encourage those who are considering using teledentistry to start locally and offer this service within their community. By taking this approach, the provider can rest assured that should providers identify the need for an in-person visit the patient will not go uncared for.

SUMMARY

Teledentistry is not a silver bullet, and it will not necessarily work for all populations or all scenarios. However, when our patients cannot get to us, we need to go to our patients. In some situations, such as those described in the current article, physically sending dentists to patients may not be the most efficient option. Therefore, to effectively meet patients' needs in ways that encourage the entire dental team to work at the top of their scope, teledentistry must fill a role that other health care delivery systems do not offer. In the current article, we have provided some background about teledentistry, including key considerations to make teledentistry successful. Examples of different models used by the dental team at coauthor Dr. Fukuoka's practice illustrate the various methods available to dental teams to address the oral health needs of patients with SHCN. Our article only scratches the surface of how our profession can use technology to connect with our patients. Because technology is rapidly advancing, it is crucial that we, as oral health providers, use the available technology in ways that place our patients in the center of our care models.

CLINICS CARE POINTS

- Teledentistry is useful to connect patients in one location to providers in a different location
- Teledentistry services must be equivalent to in-person services
- Dentists must have a trusting relationship with the individual who is collecting digital records and these individuals should be calibrated and trained on data collection; nondentists can be trained to accurately collect these records
- Checklists are helpful to ensure necessary data are collected
- Digital records possess key qualities: Teeth must be dry, all necessary anatomic landmarks should be captured, and multiple views may be required.
- Digital records can consist of multiple modalities, including photos and videos
- Ensure technology is HIPAA compliant
- Teledentistry can be useful locally
- Teledentistry has numerous applications, including but not limited to GOH, dental screenings, and dental examinations
- Be familiar with state laws pertinent to teledentistry; state laws may vary
- State laws should avoid being prescriptive so as not to tie the hands of dental providers wanting to use teledentistry
- Teledentistry examinations can lay an important foundation for the in-person visit

DISCLOSURE

Dr S.E.I. Howell is a clinical advisor for MouthWatch, LLC. He has not received any financial benefits for writing this article. Dr B. Fukuoka has financial relationships with Elevate Oral Care, MouthWatch, and Delta Dental of Idaho. She has not received any financial benefits for writing this article.

REFERENCES

1. Centers for Disease Control and Prevention. Older adult oral health: facts about older adult oral health.; 2021. Available at: https://www.cdc.gov/oralhealth/basics/adult-oral-health/adult_older.htm. Accessed July 18, 2021.
2. Bandeen-Roche K, Seplaki CL, Huang J, et al. Frailty in older adults: a nationally representative profile in the United States. J Gerontol A Biol Sci Med Sci 2015;70:1427–34.

3. Chronic diseases in America. centers for disease control and prevention. 2021. Available at: https://www.cdc.gov/chronicdisease/resources/infographic/chronic-diseases.htm. . Accessed July 18, 2021.
4. Centers for Disease Control and Prevention 2020. Disability impacts all of us Available at: https://www.cdc.gov/ncbddd/disabilityandhealth/infographic-disability-impacts-all.html. Accessed July 18, 2021.
5. National Institute of Dental and Craniofacial Research 2018. Dental caries (tooth decay) in seniors (age 65 and over) Available at: https://www.nidcr.nih.gov/research/data-statistics/dental-caries/seniors. Accessed July 18, 2021.
6. Singh ML, Papas A. Oral implications of polypharmacy in the elderly. Dent Clin North Am 2014;58:783–96.
7. Cancer stat facts: oral cavity and pharynx cancer. national cancer institute surveillance, epidemiology, and end results program. Available at: https://seer.cancer.gov/statfacts/html/oralcav.html. Accessed July 18, 2021.
8. Ward LM, Cooper SA, Hughes-McCormack L, et al. Oral health of adults with intellectual disabilities: a systematic review. J Intellect Disabil Res 2019;63:1359–78.
9. Crimmins EM, Zhang Y, Saito Y. Trends over 4 decades in disability-free life expectancy in the United States. Am J Public Health 2016;106:1287–93.
10. Health Policy Institute, American Dental Association. Dentist participation in Medicaid or CHIP; 2020. Available at: https://www.ada.org/-/media/project/ada-organization/ada/ada-org/files/resources/research/hpi/hpigraphic_0820_1.pdf. Accessed February 18, 2022.
11. Oral health and well-being among seniors in the united states. health policy institute, american dental association. Available at: https://www.ada.org/~/media/ADA/Science%20and%20Research/HPI/Files/HPIgraphic_0916_2.pdf?la=en. Accessed July 18, 2021.
12. American Dental Association 2020. ADA policy on teledentistry Available at: https://www.ada.org/en/about-the-ada/ada-positions-policies-and-statements/statement-on-teledentistry. Accessed July 18, 2021.
13. Glassman P. Improving oral health using telehealth-connected teams and the virtual dental home system of care: program and policy considerations. DentaQuest parntership for oral health advancement. 2019. Available at: https://www.carequest.org/system/files/DQ_Whitepaper_Teledentistry%20%289.19%29.pdf. Accessed July 22, 2021.
14. Rocca MA, Kudryk VL, Pajak JC, et al. The evolution of a teledentistry system within the Department of Defense. Proc AMIA Symp 1999;921–4.
15. Glassman P, Harrington M, Namakian M, et al. The virtual dental home: bringing oral health to vulnerable and underserved populations. J Calif Dent Assoc 2012;40:569–77.

The Multisensory/Snoezelen Environment to Optimize the Dental Care Patient Experience

Alison Sigal, B.H. Kin, DDS, MSc (Peds Dent), FRCD(C)[a,1,*],
Michael Sigal, DDS, Dip Peds, MSc, FRCD(C)[a,1]

KEYWORDS

- Sensory • Environment • Snoezelen • Dentistry • Special needs • Multisensory

KEY POINTS

- Snoezelen is a controlled/interactive multisensory environment addressing all the senses to help control anxiety and behavior in persons with special needs.
- A dental home that feels like "home" in the community should be created to improve access to dental care for persons with special needs.
- Anecdotal evidence states that a Snoezelen environment can improve patient cooperation and behavior and reduce the need for general anesthesia and/or sedation.
- Principles of a calming environment can be applied to the clinic/hospital/other settings such as lobby/entrance, common areas, elevators, clinics, waiting areas, preadmission area, and patient rooms.

 Video content accompanies this article at http://www.dental.theclinics.com.

BACKGROUND

Oral health is considered an integral component of overall health. The oral cavity plays a prominent role in an individual's quality of life as it pertains to communication, nutrition, emotional expression, taste, social appearance, and self-esteem.[1,2] Unfortunately, for over 30 years, dental care has been identified and continues to be recognized as one of the greatest unmet health needs facing persons with disabilities.[2–4] This apparent lack of access to oral health care is thought to be due in part to dentists' lack of knowledge, experience, and a presumed requirement of special equipment or facilities for the treatment of this population.[5] However, another factor

[a] Little Bird Pediatric Dentistry
[1] Present address: 345 Steeles Avenue East, Unit 200, Milton, Ontario, L9T3G6.
* Corresponding author.
E-mail address: alison@littlebirddental.ca

Dent Clin N Am 66 (2022) 209–228
https://doi.org/10.1016/j.cden.2021.12.001
0011-8532/22/© 2021 Elsevier Inc. All rights reserved.

that must be acknowledged is the level of dental fear or anxiety that deters this population from scheduling dental appointments or being able to cooperate for dental care.[6,7] One aspect that is within the control of the provider that may aid in reducing anxiety and possibly improving patient care is a modification of the working environment.

THE POWER OF THE ENVIRONMENT

El Marsafawy and Hesham[8] defined the environment as the physical space, people, furnishings, equipment, and actions within a space. The investigators stated that environments are living, dynamic systems that can support or hinder our activities and affect how we look, feel, and act at all times.

The power of the environment has been described by Dilts[9] as a pyramid of neurologic levels where the environment represents the foundation on which the sequential levels built upon are an individual's beliefs, values, thoughts, attitude, and behavior as the ultimate peak. Behavior as it relates to dentistry would include patient cooperation, provision of care, and of course, overall experience for all those involved.[10,11]

Dilani[12] in 2001 stated the physical environment affects our behavior, and well-designed and positively experienced environments enhance the ability to cope with stress. We react constructively and find better ways to resolve problems if we have a good experience in our surroundings.[12]

HOW DO WE SENSE OUR ENVIRONMENTS?

We use all 5 senses (hear, smell, sight, touch, taste as applicable) to become acquainted with the physical world, and as we become familiar with our surroundings, our senses convey to us all the information while our brains create significance of this information.[8]

It is widely accepted that unfamiliarity can instill anxiety, stress, and fear.[13] Norton-Westwood[14] in 2009 described unfamiliar environments or situations, common in the medical world, can lead individuals to experience intense feelings of stress and anxiety. The investigators specifically described the dentistry setting with "sterile smell of anesthetic, clay models, prophy paste, high pitched sound of drills, large cold grey leather chairs and stainless-steel instruments with various 'torture like' ends.[14] As such, what is of utmost importance is to create a sense of familiarity in the environment, where changing the design of the environment with the patient in mind can positively influence patient outcome.[15]

Melmed[16] in 2001 demonstrated positive environments resulted in the subject's attention being focused intently on the surrounding stimuli providing an altered state with a concomitant reduction of awareness of discomforting or nocuous stimuli, when compared with dull environments, which force us to turn to our inner selves as the exterior provides no stimulation, which can lead to increased anxiety, fear, and distress.[17]

Vuong and colleagues[18] in 2008 investigated the design and impact of the waiting room specifically because it represents the first interaction point between users (patients) and the environment. The investigators perceived impact expressed through 3 categories: emotive, cognitive, and associative responses. Data revealed people mainly speak about environment concepts and the impact of the designs as they related to their feelings (eg, I would feel okay sitting and waiting) with most individuals expressing preference for rooms that *felt* like home, which was associated with reduced anxiety, stress, and improved calmness.[18]

INTRODUCTION TO SNOEZELEN AND SENSORY INTEGRATION

Being able to control and interact with your environment is the major aspect of feeling at home, which is important for feeling comfortable and is the premise behind Snoezelen.[19]

Snoezelen was developed in Holland in the 1970s as a controlled/interactive multisensory environment where as many of the 5 senses are addressed in the preference/power/control of the individual. This environment was first explored with individuals with anxiety and those with intellectual disabilities, resulting in consistent reductions of the individual's anxiety, providing an increased sense of calm and comfort. A Snoezelen environment therefore can be defined as a multisensory adapted environment coupled with patient-centered therapy.[20,21]

A Snoezelen environment may include having a partially lit room with special lighting effects, relaxing music, vibration, or aromas. Shapiro and colleagues[22] in 2001 incorporated these environmental attributes when providing dental care and found this reduced pain and maladaptive behaviors, enhanced behavior facilitation, and balanced heart rate (objective indicator of anxiety).

Shapiro and colleagues[23] in 2007 conducted a random crossover design with 19 patients (ages 6–11 year old) to determine if a Snoezelen environment could affect behavior in the dental setting. The investigators measured their anxiety through questionnaire and observation before care; then half received dental recalls with Snoezelen conditions (SC) or regular conditions (RC) with crossover after 4 months. During the appointment, electrodermal activity was monitored (a measure of relaxation versus arousal). Snoezelen conditions included visual sensation (adapted, dimmed, color effects with solar projector), auditory and somatosensory (rhythmic music with vibration on dental chair), and tactile stimulation (lead apron cover for a deep hugging pressure effect). Results revealed that the mean duration and magnitude of anxious behavior was significantly reduced in the SC versus regular conditions, and 80% of the patients preferred the SC conditions.[23]

A modified sensory environment such as Snoezelen can result in a subject's attention being focused intently on the positive stimuli, causing an altered state with a concomitant reduction in awareness of discomforting or nocuous stimuli.[16]

At present, multisensory controlled environments and associated equipment are widely commercially available, however, only the multisensory resources provided by Flaghouse can be referred to as Snoezelen.

OUR COMMUNITY PRACTICE: LITTLE BIRD PEDIATRIC DENTISTRY DESIGN

Having previously worked within a hospital environment providing care for patients of all ages with special needs, the creation of Little Bird Pediatric Dentistry in 2016 came from the author's' desire to build a community practice for persons with special needs of all ages, focused on the positive power of environment and Snoezelen/sensory integration. The objective was to create a clinic that fosters the feelings of home and comfort, with the goal of improving patient care and experience.

Understanding the significance of environment, one must recognize there are several "environments" experienced in the course of a patient's appointment, and each contributes to their ultimate behavior/cooperation and experience, from their arrival, parking, and entry to the provision of their dental care and departure. The goal must be to minimize any potential stressors that are within our control at each point, in the hope of providing the best patient experience.

Highlighted in the following discussion are various important design features present at Little Bird Pediatric Dentistry that incorporate the principles of Snoezelen and patient-centered care alongside rationale for added insight.

PATIENT ARRIVAL AND PARKING

- Having a fully accessible building (parking lot, ramps, main entrance, washroom)

Several buildings unfortunately are missing one or several of these essential items. For persons with special needs and their caregivers/families, ensuring their arrival does not evoke unnecessary stress is invaluable.

- Elevator

The elevator represents an enclosed moving space that can be a source of anxiety. A sensory tile should be installed (**Fig. 1**), something that is interactive and can serve as a focal point of distraction. Distraction outward reduces internal stress.

- Hallways or main corridors

From a design perspective seeing or walking down an empty hallway can provoke notable anxiety through measured elevated blood pressure, heart rate, and respiratory rate. Instead, sensory tiles should be installed ideally with an element of patient interaction/control along the walls to act as distraction or focal points to focus on (**Fig. 2**).

ALL SPACES AND CLINICAL ROOMS

- Adjustable lighting (dimmers)

Traditionally, medical environments are known for having bright, florescent overhead lights; this can be a trigger or source of anxiety for individuals. Having the ability to adjust the lighting to best suit the patient is essential. In most of our spaces the lights are either off or notably dimmed for maximal patient relaxation and comfort. See **Fig. 3** for provision of dental care at Little Bird in a dimmed setting.

- Natural light (windows)

Vuong and colleagues[18] in 2008 noted natural lighting was one of 3 elements most discussed in relation to patient comfort in a space. Little Bird has a minimum of 1 window in every operatory/space to allow for maximal natural light. Each window also has adjustable blinds to control as needed.[18]

- Adjustable overhead music (volume control)

Cunningham and colleagues[24] in 1997 demonstrated music can touch patients deeply and thus transform their anxiety and stress into relaxation and healing. Most beneficial responses for patients, however, are elicited when the music is familiar, desirable, and meaningful to them. Standley[25] concluded that the use

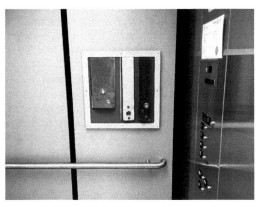

Fig. 1. Tactile sensory interactive panel installed within elevator.

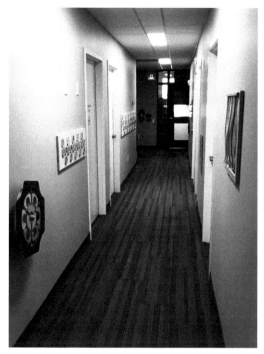

Fig. 2. Tactile sensory interactive tiles installed throughout the main hallway.

of music in dental studies may have an audioanalgesic response because of several different factors including the direct neurologic suppression of pain, masking of sound, and distraction.[26] Inquiring about patient preference or desire to be louder, quieter, or off is important.

- Olfactory/smell: fragrance-free environment

Several studies have revealed effects of odors on cognition, emotion, mood, and memory.[27] Although fragrances have the ability to trigger positive emotion, this is highly variable based on personal preference, culture, and past experience. To avoid eliciting negative feelings, emotion, and/or allergic reactions, it is best

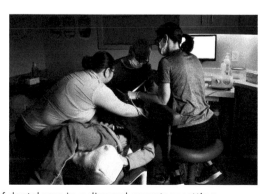

Fig. 3. Provision of dental care in a dimmed operatory setting.

to provide a neutral fragrance-free environment (eg, avoiding perfumes or colognes, scent misters).
- Visual: soft wall colors

Soft neutral colors such as cream, blue, and yellow to minimize extraneous ambient energy.

WAITING AREA/CALMING AND PRIVATE ROOMS

- Visual and somatosensory: ball bubble tube (**Fig. 4**)

Continual flow of bubbles and balls floating from base to top and returning is mesmerizing to the eye, and also provides a subtle vibration to the touch. A sturdy box around the base allows for patients to stand, sit, hug, and touch this bubble tube for added comfort.
- Personal space and various areas/zones

El Marsafawy and Hesham[8] explained that to improve patient comfort, waiting room layouts should have variety. The layout should allow for families/groups to sit together; have single chairs, not facing each other; and ensure that chairs have armrests, as lack of personal space is a primary patient complaint and armrests can define a designated personal space.[8]

At Little Bird, our waiting area contains comfortable chairs, rocking chairs, a quiet reading couch for families, stools surrounding provided tablets, floor pillows for younger patient tablet use and an interactive sensory area (**Fig. 5**). There are ample paths surrounding our waiting area in addition to private calming rooms for patients who desire to walk and explore, which is encouraged.
- Tactile stimulation (liquid tiles, Sound Shell Chair)

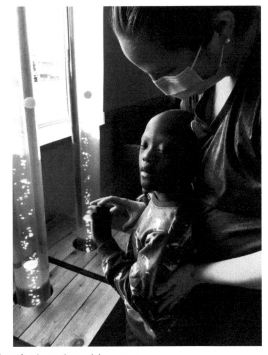

Fig. 4. Ball bubble tube in main waiting area.

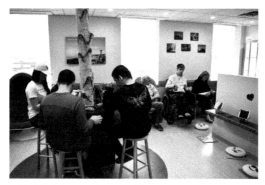

Fig. 5. Waiting room highlighting various settings.

Liquid tiles contain colors that (**Fig. 6**) with any pressure (touch, step, and so forth) mix and move. These tiles are strategically placed within the waiting area and throughout the entire clinic, acting as focal points to lead the patient to desired destination points.

The Sound Shell Chair (**Fig. 7**) represents a Flaghouse Snoezelen soft-cushioned chair that incorporates music and vibration. The shape and construction make

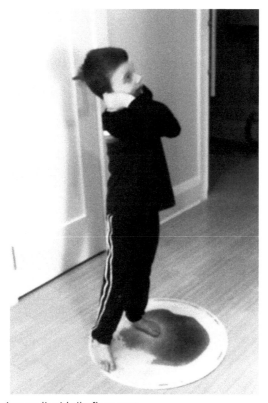

Fig. 6. Patient playing on liquid tile floor mat.

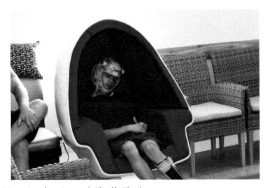

Fig. 7. Patient waiting in the Sound Shell Chair.

it perfect for both sound isolation and acoustics. The chamberlike shape and up-holstered interior cancel out most outside noise, providing a unique environment for meditation and relaxation.

- Auditory (waterfall feature: see **Fig. 8**)

The sound of natural flowing water is one of the best sound diffusers, which is very beneficial in a dental office to help cancel the sounds generated by high-pitch drills to assist in reducing this potential stressor. Flowing water is also a sound that commonly elicits calmness and relaxation, regularly featured in places of mediation. At Little Bird our floor-to-ceiling waterfall feature can be heard throughout the clinic and is also interactive, allowing for patient touch.

- Interactive (ball wall, sensory tiles)

Having screen-free activities for engagement and enjoyment; various textures, sounds, racing balls through a loopy wall-mounted panel (**Fig. 9**), and with each patient action, there is a reaction.

- Private patient calming and/or waiting rooms with couches (before/after appointment)

At Little Bird we feature 2 rooms (**Fig. 10**) referred to as our Space room and Under-water room. Space room (**Fig. 11**) has a laser stars projector mounted, aimed to-ward the ceiling and with space design features. Closure of the pocket door to this room, transforms the space into a galaxy far away. With adjustable lighting and music, this can also be controlled to suit patient desires.

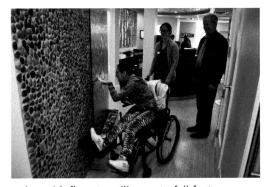

Fig. 8. Patient interacting with floor-to-ceiling waterfall feature.

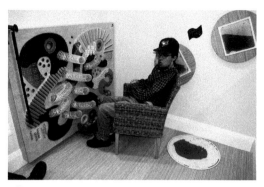

Fig. 9. Loopy Ball Wall in main waiting area.

The Underwater room (**Fig. 12**) is located behind the waterfall, where the flowing water creates a natural shimmer throughout the room, and the design is augmented with underwater-friendly decals. Closure of the pocket door allows for patient privacy and relaxation.

To view a video taken of the main waiting room area highlighting many of the items listed and described earlier please view Video 1.

OPERATORIES

- Ceiling-mounted TV with Netflix (above dental chair)

Allowing for the patients to select a program that brings them happiness will aid in distraction (**Fig. 13**).

- Availability of weighted blankets

These blankets are used for comfort as well as gentle protective stabilization. Ideally they have Velcro closure. These blankets are available at Little Bird in various weights and styles (mesh vs solid).

- Initial consultation room to be as neutral as possible

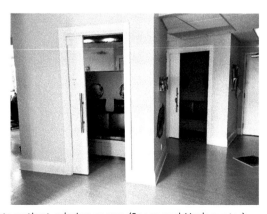

Fig. 10. Two private patient-calming rooms (Space and Underwater).

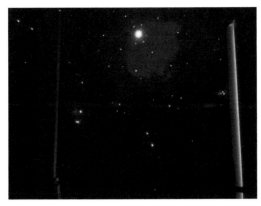

Fig. 11. Laser stars projection within space room when door is closed.

At Little Bird our initial consultation or new patient examination areas have no visible medical or dental items. Instead they feature various sensory items from liquid floor tiles to wall-mounted sensory interactive panels, in themes of the beach or the mountains, to be able to build a relationship and gain patient trust and comfort before conducting a dental examination.

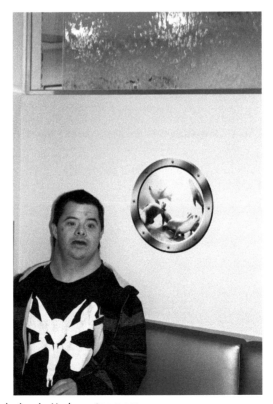

Fig. 12. Patient relaxing in Underwater room.

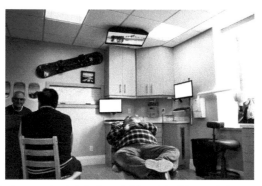

Fig. 13. Patient relaxing on dental chair watching television gaining comfort in space.

PANOREX ROOM

- Window facing, side entry, and mirror (**Fig. 14**A and B)

Most dental offices have their panorex or radiograph rooms built as small, enclosed spaces where patients are typically facing a wall and asked to remain still for their image, which can be a notable trigger for anxiety.

At Little Bird, the panorex room is designed for the patient to face a large window, looking outside, providing the sense of openness and ample focal points of distraction (eg, cars, people, changing seasons). The panorex itself is a side-entry machine that is accessible, allowing image capture for those in wheelchairs or using assisted devices.

We also have a mirror situated to allow for patients, especially those who are hearing impaired, to be able to see our clinical staff taking the image to be able to communicate through body language so they are aware of image status.

SNOEZELEN TREATMENT ROOM

- Bubble wall with interactive color changing (**Figs. 15** and **16**)

Visual feature with the constant floating bubbles from floor to ceiling and interactive with a control panel, which allows for patients to change the color of the bubbles. This feature also has a vibrational feel to the touch and relaxing flowing water sound.

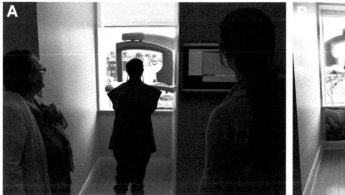
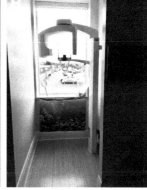

Fig. 14. (*A*) Patient having panorex image taken highlighting design features of panorex room. (*B*) Panorex room, side entry-accessible panorex.

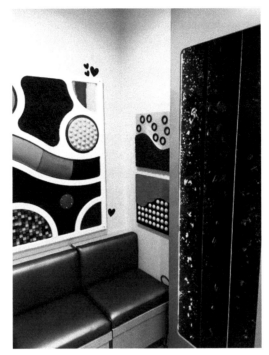

Fig. 15. Snoezelen treatment room.

- Liquid floor tiles, sensory wall-mounted panels, and tactile items

All sensory based, with various textures and interactions to evoke fun and interaction.

- Comfortable custom bench/couch seating and is fully accessible
- Hidden (pocket door) mobile dental unit (**Fig. 17**)

This unit allows for the initial patient meeting, discussion, and history taking to feel comfortable and at ease, and allows the patient to interact and enjoy all sensory items present in the space. When care is to be provided, the innocuous mobile dental unit is

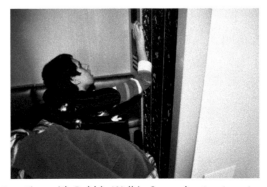

Fig. 16. Patient interacting with Bubble Wall in Snoezelen treatment room.

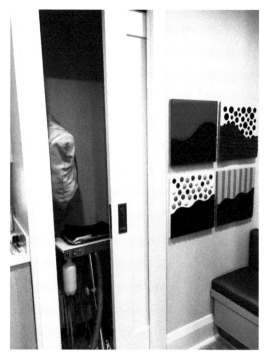

Fig. 17. Hidden mobile dental cart within Snoezelen treatment room.

rolled out, and we are able to provide care in a space where the patient already feels grounded and comfortable.

CLASSROOM/PRE-OPERATIVE ROOM FOR GENERAL ANESTHESIA CARE

- Projector with Netflix or nature scenes such as rolling ocean waves (**Fig. 18**)
- Trampoline: rebounding therapy

Trampoline bouncing can induce relaxation and release stress and anxiety.[28] At Little Bird, we have 2 Health Bounce B-Pods, which are rebounder devices (trampolines)

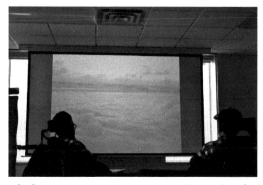

Fig. 18. Patients enjoying ocean waves on a projector in the classroom before appointments.

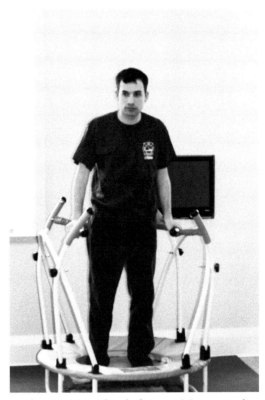

Fig. 19. Patient rebounding on trampoline before receiving general anesthesia care.

that feature a padded C-frame handle for upper body support providing additional stability and safety. Patients may use these trampolines (**Fig. 19**) before or after their appointments to enhance their overall experience by reducing any preoperative or postoperative nervous energy/anxiety and providing a sense of enjoyment/fun. With less patient anxiety or stress, you increase the likelihood of increased patient cooperation and compliance.

To view a video taken of one of our patients enjoying the rebounding trampoline before their dental appointment please view Video 2.

OPERATORY SET UP FOR PROVISION OF GENERAL ANESTHESIA CARE

- Room connection with Snoezelen room: sensory tiles and bubble wall feature
- Ceiling-mounted television with Netflix show of patient preference
- Weighted blanket as requested for patient comfort
- Adjustable lights and room music (typically dimmed and low volume)
- Parents or support workers present at time of induction for added comfort
- Inhalational induction (as opposed to intravenous) unless requested

Fig. 20 shows our patient after rebounding, calmly receiving his inhalational induction.

Note: Little Bird Pediatric Dentistry Clinic is a recipient of Snoezelen materials from Flaghouse, global experts and leaders in Snoezelen.

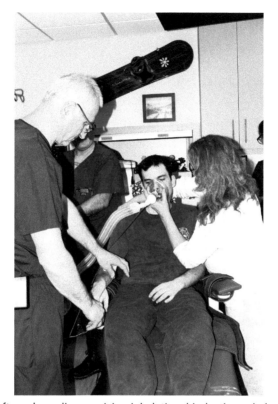

Fig. 20. Patient after rebounding receiving inhalational induction calmly.

LITTLE BIRD PEDIATRIC DENTISTRY PATIENT CARE OUTCOMES

Patients with special needs previously seen in a regional hospital dental clinic are much more cooperative and relaxed for care provided at Little Bird Pediatric Dentistry with more treatment being provided with local measures only. As of March 2019, 37

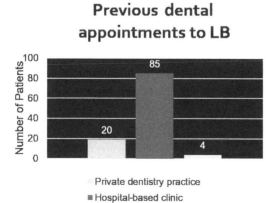

Fig. 21. Graph of previous dental appointments to Little Bird (LB).

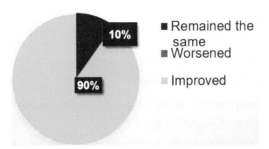

Fig. 22. Visit at Little Bird compared with previous dental and/or medical appointments.

patients of 710 (5.2%) were identified to still need general anesthesia for provision of their dental needs when compared with the hospital records where 50% of this patient base required general anesthesia. From more than 700 persons with special needs seen within the first 1.5 years of Little Bird being open, 109 randomly selected patient feedback surveys were reviewed following their new patient examination at Little Bird. The majority (85%) of patients surveyed were previously seen at a hospital-based clinic (**Fig. 21**), and 90% stated that compared with their previous dental and/or medical appointments, patient care/cooperation/experience was improved at Little Bird (**Fig. 22**). When asked which factors they thought contributed to the improved experience, 98% stated the Little Bird environment and staff approach to care were the primary factors (**Fig. 23**).

In regard to how the respondents would rank the patient's overall experience on a numerical scale, the majority (61%) stated 10 of 10, as best experience ever (**Fig. 24**).

From the patient perspective, there is an overwhelming component to care in a routine hospital-based setting. The regional hospital that included an associated

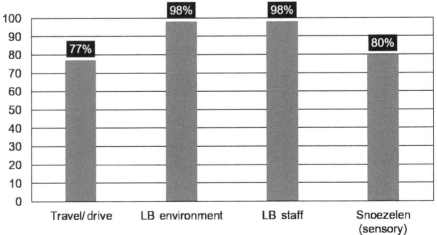

Fig. 23. Contributing factors to improved patient experience at Little Bird (LB).

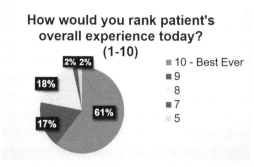

How would you rank patient's overall experience today? (1-10)

- 10 - Best Ever
- 9
- 8
- 7
- 5

Fig. 24. Patient's overall ranking of experience at Little Bird.

dental clinic and facilities to provide care under general anesthesia was considerably more intimidating than a community-based dental clinic designed to provide a sense of calming. Consider the registration and admission process followed by the preoperative preparation area with all the other patients at the hospital after which the patient must enter an operating room/surgical suite that by design is multipurpose for all the various surgical specialties. This is then followed by a communal recovery area again with traditional bays with other patients and staff until discharge. The actual anesthesia and dental care provided to the individual with special needs may be the same in both venues, but the community environment has an inherent calming influence on the patient, which facilitates the provision of more extensive dental care without the need for sedation. Furthermore, for those who still required care under general anesthesia they were more relaxed and cooperative for the induction of anesthesia in the calming environment. In the hospital setting there was a greater reliance on protective stabilization, many times with security and the use of preoperative sedation to assist with induction of anesthesia than at the community clinic. One could suggest the creation of a calming environment within a hospital setting could have similar positive effects on patient's behavior and cooperation.

Family, caregivers and patient satisfaction at Little Bird is very high, and feedback has been positive; 91% noticed improvement in patient cooperation, and 95% agreed the environment made a difference in the patient's behavior (eg, reduced agitation levels, improved relaxation, engagement, and happiness). **Figs. 25 and 26** show Drs. Alison and Michael Sigal providing care at Little Bird Pediatric Dentistry.

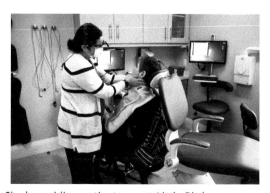

Fig. 25. Dr. Alison Sigal providing patient care at Little Bird.

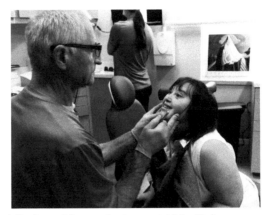

Fig. 26. Dr. Michael Sigal providing patient care at Little Bird.

General anesthesia provided to patients with special needs at Little Bird compared with previous hospital ambulatory surgery experiences with Dr Michael Sigal:

- Patients are more cooperative and compliant.
- No provision of preoperative sedative agents are necessary.
- There is a reduced need for stabilization for inhalational induction.
- Feedback from caregivers and families is very positive; they are regularly astonished at the difference from previous hospital general anesthetic experiences.

SUMMARY

Creation of a comfort-oriented, homelike dental environment using Snoezelen multisensory themed interactive devices can play a vital role in fostering positive behaviors expressed by persons with special needs. Anecdotal evidence strongly suggests that persons with special needs are calmer and more receptive for dental care without the need for sedation or general anesthesia when introduced to care in this type of environment. A calming multisensory environment has the promise to reduce fear and anxiety, which should improve the overall experience and cooperation of the individual. Hopefully that the creation of more clinical spaces that include a neurosensory interactive environment will have the potential to improve their access to needed dental care due to improved, predictable behavior.

CLINICS CARE POINTS

- The environment is key to how we feel in any given space and can help to facilitate a positive dental care experience.
- A calming environment in which the individual has some level of control may have the ability to reduce anxiety and improve behavior and cooperation in preparation for dental care.
- Dental clinics (all health care clinics) should focus on creating a calming environment, which can improve behavior and thus lead to improved access to dental care in the community setting for persons with special needs.
- Snoezelen was developed by the Dutch in the 1970s to seek, explore, and relax by addressing all the human senses in a controlled environment.

DISCLOSURE

Dr. A. Sigal: Founder, owner, practitioner, and researcher at Little Bird Pediatric Dentistry (community private practice); founder and president (2008–2020): Federal Non-Profit Organization, Oral Health, Total Health. Little Bird Pediatric Dentistry Clinic is a recipient of Snoezelen Materials from Flaghouse, global experts and leaders in Snoezelen. Dr. M. Sigal: Pediatric Dentist at Little Bird Pediatric Dentistry (community private practice) and professor emeritus Pediatric Dentistry, University of Toronto.

ACKNOWLEDGEMENTS

The authors like to extend sincere thanks and gratitude to Rebecca Robertson, who assisted with data collection, photography and preparation of content for this publication.

SUPPLEMENTARY DATA

Supplementary data related to this article can be found online at doi:10.1016/j.cden.2021.12.001.

REFERENCES

1. Stiefel DJ. Delivery of dental care to the disabled. J Can Dent Assoc 1981;47: 657–62.
2. Sigal A, Sigal MJ. Overview of a hospital based dental programme for persons with special needs. J Disabil Oral Health 2006;7:176–84.
3. Levine N, Sigal M, Pulver F. Dentistry for the disabled. Ontario Dentist 1986; 63(6):14–9.
4. Newacheck P, McManus M, Fox H, et al. Access to health care for children with special health care needs. Paediatrics 2000;105:760–6.
5. Waldman H, Perlman S. Why is providing dental care to people with mental retardation and other developmental disabilities such a low priority? Public Health Rep 2002;117:435–40.
6. Martin M, Kinoshita-Byrne J, Getz T. Dental fear in a special needs clinic population of persons with disabilities. Spec Care Dentist 2002;22:99–102. https://doi.org/10.1111/j.1754-4505.2002.tb01170.x.
7. Gordon SM, Dionne RA, Snyder J. Dental fear and anxiety as a barrier to accessing oral health care among patients with special health care needs. Spec Care Dentistry 1998;18:88–92. https://doi.org/10.1111/j.1754-4505.1998.tb00910.x.
8. El Marsafawy Hesham. Design for effective and affective medical environments. Thesis Publication; 2006. University of Duisburg-Essen, Germany.
9. Dilts R. Changing belief systems with NLP. Cupertino, (CA): Meta Publications; 1990. p. 1–68.
10. Sandu A. Using the Pyramid of Neurological Levels in the Human Resources Motivation Management. Revista Romaneasca pentru Educatie Multidimensionala 2016;8(2):31–44. https://doi.org/10.18662/rrem/2016.0802.03.
11. Lane RD. Levels of emotional awareness: Neurological, psychological, and social perspectives. In: Bar-On R, Parker JDA, editors. The handbook of emotional intelligence: Theory, development, assessment, and application at home, school, and in the workplace. Jossey-Bass; 2000. p. 171–91.
12. Dilani A. Psychosocially supportive design- Scandinavian healthcare design. The result of the 2nd International Conference on design and health organized by the

Karolinska Institute in Stockholm. Stockholm: AB Svensk Byggtjanst; 2001. p. 31–7.

13. Frumkin H. Healthy places: exploring the evidence. Am J Public Health 2003; 93(9):1451–6.

14. Norton-Westwood D, Pearson A, Roberstson-Malt S. The ability of environmental healthcare design strategies to impact event related anxiety in pediatric patients: a comprehensive review. University of Adelaide; 2009. Joanna Briggs Institute, Adelaide.

15. Ulrich R. View through a window may influence recovery from surgery. Science 1984;224(4647):420.

16. Melmed R. Mind, body & medicine: an integrative text. New York: Oxford University Press; 2001. p. 362–86.

17. Mahnke F. Color, environment and human response: an interdisciplinary understanding of colour and its use as a beneficial element in the design of the architectural environment. USA: Van Nostrand: a division of International Thomson Publishing Inc.; 1996.

18. Vuong K, Cain R, Burton E, et al. The impact of healthcare waiting environment design on end-user perception and well being. Engineering and Physical Science Research Council (EPSRC); 2008. University of Warwick, Coventry United Kingdom.

19. Dovey K. Home and homelessness. Home environments. New York and London: Plenum Press; 1985. p. 33–64.

20. Hulsegge J, Verheul A. Snoezelen: Another world. Chesterfield: Rompa; 1987.

21. Patterson I. Snoezelen as a casual leisure activity for people with a developmental disability. Therapeutic Recreation Journal; 2004. ProQuest Education Journals 2004;38–43. Pg. 289 -300.

22. Shapiro M, Roth D, Marcus A, et al. The effect of lighting on children with developmental disabilities. J Int Spec Needs Education 2001;4:19–23.

23. Shapiro M, Melmed RN, Sgan-Cohen HD, et al. Behavioral and physiological effect of dental environment sensory adaptation on children's dental anxiety. Eur J Oral Sci 2007;115:479–83.

24. Cunningham MF, Monson B, Bookbinder M, et al. Introducing a music program in the perioperative area. AORN 1997;66(4):674–81.

25. Standley JM. Music research in medical/dental treatment: meta-analysis and clinical applications. J Music Ther 1986;23(2):65–122. https://doi.org/10.1093/jmt/23.2.56.

26. Biley F. Effects on patient well-being of music listening as a nursing intervention. J Clin Nurs 2000;9:668–77.

27. Lorig T. Human EEG and odor response. Prog Neurobiol 1989;33:387–98.

28. Carter A. Rebounder & stress relief. 2017. Available at. https://rebound-air.com/stress-relief-best-rebounders/. 23 June 2021.

Thinking Outside the Tooth

Diagnosis and Management of Patients with Neuropathic Orofacial Pain

Akihiro Ando, DDS[a,b], Phuu P. Han, DDS, PhD[c],*,
Seena Patel, DMD, MPH[d,e]

KEYWORDS

- Neuropathic pain • Trigeminal neuralgia • Trigeminal neuropathy • Red flags
- Orofacial pain

KEY POINTS

- Orofacial pain in the absence of pathologic condition in the dentition and the surrounding tissues can pose a significant challenge to dentists and patients.
- Neuropathic orofacial pain is a pathologic pain owing to a lesion or dysfunction of the nervous system, and the severity of pain is irrelevant to the proportion of tissue injury.
- Thorough and systematic pain history taking and recognition of red flags are crucial in the diagnosis and management of patients presenting with perplexing orofacial pain.
- Reassess and refer the patient to specialists, such as orofacial pain specialists, endodontists, or neurologists, when the pain is refractory to traditional dental treatments.
- Accurate and timely diagnosis and treatment are vital to prevent unnecessary procedures and to prevent a delay in diagnosis of a serious underlying disease.

Abbreviations	
TN	trigeminal Neuralgia
PTTN	posttraumatic Trigeminal Neuropathy
PIFP	persistent Idiopathic Facial Pain
BMS	burning Mouth Syndrome
ICOP	international Classification of Orofacial Pain
ICHD-3	international Classification of Headache Disorders
VZV	varicella Zoster Virus

[a] Ando Orofacial Pain and Oral Medicine Clinic, 8-12-8 Todoroki Setagaya-ku, Tokyo, 158-0082, Japan; [b] Showa University School of Dentistry, 1-5-8 Hatanodai Shinagawa-ku, Tokyo 142-8555, Japan; [c] Garvey Dental Group, 9866 Garvey Ave, Suite A, El Monte, CA 91733, USA; [d] Arizona School of Dentistry and Oral Health, Advanced Care Center, A.T. Still University, 5835 East Still Circle, Mesa, AZ 85206, USA; [e] Southwest Orofacial Group, 10214 North Tatum Blvd, Suite A-1100, Phoenix, AZ 85028, USA
* Corresponding author.
E-mail address: phuuhan@hotmail.com

Dent Clin N Am 66 (2022) 229–244
https://doi.org/10.1016/j.cden.2022.01.003
0011-8532/22/© 2022 Elsevier Inc. All rights reserved.

INTRODUCTION

Oral health care providers are often the first-line practitioners to diagnose a patient's pain in the orofacial region. At times, they will encounter patients who present with a perplexing type of orofacial pain that occurs in the absence of any organic pathologic condition affecting the dentition and the surrounding structures. These types of pain can pose a significant challenge to both the clinician and the patient. They are usually chronic, and the source of pain is often difficult to locate and diagnose. The initial step in diagnosing any chronic orofacial pain is to first rule out odontogenic sources of pain[1] (ie, pulpal, hyperocclusion, cracked tooth). Then, the clinician should consider the various nonodontogenic sources of orofacial pain, which include musculoskeletal, neurovascular, and/or neuropathic types of pain.[2] In this article, the authors focus on the diagnosis of neuropathic orofacial pains. They review how to take a thorough pain history, the "red flags" of orofacial pain, and the diagnosis, evaluation, and management of each type of trigeminal neuropathic pain.

When describing the types of pain, the International Association for the Study of Pain defines 2 important terms: nociceptive and neuropathic pain.[3] Nociceptive pain results from the stimulation of the nociceptors throughout the body in response to actual tissue damage (nonneural tissue). Nociceptive pain is a protective type of pain that occurs in response to tissue injury and is considered to be a physiologic pain.[2] Neuropathic pain, on the other hand, is initiated by a primary lesion or dysfunction of the nerve and is a pathologic pain.[3] The nerve lesion or dysfunction leads to phenotypic changes in the nervous system, and patients with neuropathic pain can experience paradoxic sensory perceptions (**Box 1**), spontaneous ongoing or shooting pain, and exaggerated pain responses to both noxious and nonnoxious stimuli.[3,4]

Box 1
Examples of paradoxic sensory perceptions[3,4]

Negative sensation
Hypoesthesia: Decreased sensitivity to stimulation, excluding the special senses. For example, reduced perception or numbness when touching or stroking the skin with a cotton swab

Spontaneous/evoked abnormal sensation
Paresthesia: An abnormal sensation, whether spontaneous or evoked but not unpleasant. For example, tingling sensation

Positive/exaggerated unpleasant sensation
Dysesthesia: An unpleasant, abnormal sensation, whether spontaneous or evoked. A dysesthesia is always unpleasant. Hyperalgesia and allodynia are special cases of dysesthesia. Hyperalgesia: Increased pain from a stimulus that normally provokes pain, that is, increased pain on suprathreshold stimulation.
For example, pricking the skin with a sharp stick produced exaggerated pain response Allodynia: Pain owing to a stimulus that does not normally evoke pain. Allodynia means there is pain upon stimulation by a nonpainful stimulus.
For example, stroking the skin with a cotton swab causes pain; percussion pain on otherwise healthy teeth

Data from International Association for the Study of Pain. IASP Taxonomy Working Group. Part III Pain Terms: A current list with definitions and notes on usage (Updated 2011) Available at https://www.iasp-pain.org/wp-content/uploads/2021/07/Part_III-PainTerms.pdf Accessed on Aug 26, 2021 and Baron R, Binder A, Wasner G. Neuropathic pain: diagnosis, pathophysiological mechanisms, and treatment. Lancet Neurol. 2010;9(8):807-19.

Depending on the nature and duration of the pain, orofacial neuropathic pain can be further categorized into continuous or episodic types. Continuous forms of neuropathic pain include posttraumatic trigeminal neuropathy (PTTN), persistent idiopathic facial pain (PIFP), burning mouth syndrome (BMS), and postherpetic neuralgia. The episodic neuropathic pains occur in the form of neuralgia, such as trigeminal neuralgia (TN), glossopharyngeal neuralgia, geniculate neuralgia, and superior laryngeal neuralgia.[5–7]

Pain History

When evaluating a patient with neuropathic orofacial pain, it is critical to obtain a detailed pain history. Focusing on key pain characteristics can aid the clinician in detecting "red flags" that could be indicative of a more ominous diagnosis. Unfortunately, most patients will not provide a detailed account of their pain. Therefore, clinicians need to know what to ask. Using a systematic approach to this history-taking makes it easy and efficient to determine the necessary aspects of pain.

First, the orofacial pain history should include detailed aspects of the patient's pain complaints (**Box 2**).[8]

Clarifying the onset of the pain helps identify whether this is acute or chronic pain. Identifying any incident occurring before the pain can provide further insight to a traumatic source. The quality of pain refers to the description of the pain. The patient's description of the pain is instrumental in determining the type of orofacial pain. Neuropathic pain may be described as aching, dull, sharp, throbbing, burning, stinging, shooting, electrical, cutting, or itchy (OFP Guidelines Book).[9] Validated screening tools have been developed to help differentiate neuropathic pain from nociceptive pain, including the Leeds Assessment of Neuropathic Symptoms and Signs (LANSS and S-LANSS, the short version), Douleur Neuropathique, Neuropathic Pain Questionnaire, ID-Pain, and PainDETECT.[9]

Modifying factors to the pain help determine what makes the pain better or worse. Prior evaluation and treatments are also an important piece to the pain history. Specifically, evaluating the risk for neuropathic pain is dependent on whether the patient had a prior history of inflammatory pain preceding any dental or surgical treatment.

Box 2
Pain history[8]

Onset

Location

Frequency

Duration

Quality

Severity

Causative factors

Aggravating and ameliorating factors

Associated symptoms

Prior treatments or evaluations

Data from Bender SD. Assessment of the Orofacial Pain Patient. Dent Clin North Am. 2018;62(4):525 to 532.

Box 3
Identifying "red flags"

S: Systemic symptoms or disease

N: Neurologic signs or symptoms

O: Onset being sudden

O: Onset after age of 50 years

P (4): Pattern change (progressive, precipitants, postural aggravation, and papilledema)

Dieb and colleagues[10] found that 73% of patients with orofacial neuropathic pain reported a history of prior inflammatory pain.

Red Flags

Although it is rare (approximately 1%), the pain could be a manifestation of a significant, underlying disease.[9] Therefore, the clinician must integrate a plan to identify pain characteristics suggestive of a secondary cause ("red flags"). The most well-known, systematic approach for this uses the pneumonic: *SNOOP-4 RED FLAGS* (**Box 3**). Although this specifically targets identifying any secondary cause of headache, it can also be applied to orofacial pain. Headaches can also present in the orofacial region, which is why this pneumonic should be incorporated into the history.

S refers to identifying a systemic cause or symptom of the pain. Systemic symptoms include fever, chills, night sweats, stiff neck, myalgias, unintentional weight loss, chest pain, or shortness of breath that has accompanied the pain. Make note of a history of cancer or immunosuppressing disease. Specific systemic diseases, like giant cell arteritis, intracranial infection, or malignancy, can present as a headache and facial pain (**Box 4**).[11] In addition, ischemic cardiac disease can refer pain into the jaws,[12] and patients may describe the referred facial pain as pressure or burning that is aggravated by exertion, chest pain, and/or shortness of breath.[13]

Box 4
Systemic diseases causing facial pain

Anemia

Adrenal insufficiency

Autoimmune disease (rheumatoid arthritis, systemic lupus erythematosus, scleroderma, Sjögren syndrome)

Endocrine disorders (diabetes mellitus, Hashimoto thyroiditis)

Fibromyalgia

Giant cell arteritis

HIV/AIDS

Cardiac disease (hypertension, ischemic heart disease)

Lyme disease

Malignancy

Neurodegenerative (amyotrophic lateral sclerosis, multiple sclerosis, myasthenia gravis)

Renal failure

N refers to neurologic signs or symptoms accompanying the headache. These can be focal or global and include vision change; altered sensation; weakness; dizziness; imbalance; change in memory, personality, or behavior; paralysis; or loss of consciousness. These symptoms can be a sign of a neoplastic, inflammatory, infectious, or vascular central nervous system disorder.[11] Orofacial neurologic deficits include numbness, dysesthesia, paresthesia, facial weakness, dysphagia, hearing loss, hypoglossal nerve dysfunction, masticatory muscle weakness and fatigue, and orofacial dystonia.[12,14–16] Metastasis to the mandible, osteonecrosis of the jaws, or neuropathy owing to systemic disease can result in sensory loss to the face.[17]

The first *O* refers to the onset of the headache and how quickly a patient feels no pain at all to severe, debilitating pain. The shorter this timeframe is, the more ominous the underlying cause. In fact, a sudden-onset, severe pain in the head is considered a "red flag" until proven otherwise. Vascular crises, such as intracranial hemorrhage, cerebral infarction, cerebral venous thrombosis, and cervical artery dissection, can present with a sudden-onset headache. Examples of nonvascular disorders include high or low cerebrospinal fluid pressure, intracranial neoplasm, and intracranial infection.[9,11,12]

The second *O* refers to the onset of the headache or facial pain occurring after age 50 years.[11] Inquire if the reported headache is new or different from previous headaches experienced. New-onset primary headaches and facial pain occurring after age 50 years is unusual, and therefore, requires further evaluation.[12] Possible causes of this include intracranial neoplasm, or inflammatory or infectious central nervous system (CNS) disease. Giant cell arteritis is a vasculitis that occurs in people older than 50 years that can lead to loss of vision. It can present as a temporal headache accompanied by pain in the jaws, mimicking a temporomandibular disorder.[12]

The *P* refers to any pattern change to the headache. There are 4 features of pattern change to evaluate: progressive, precipitants, postural aggravation, and papilledema. Inquire if the headache is progressive and if there is a change in headache frequency or quality of the headache. Then, determine if there are precipitants to the headache, such as exertion or Valsalva maneuver. This can occur with Chiari malformation and cerebrospinal fluid disorders. Headaches that change with postural changes may indicate a change in cerebrospinal fluid pressure. Last, if the patient reports vision problems with the headache, there may be papilledema or swelling around the optic nerve.[9,11]

Although it is quite rare for headaches and facial pain to be due to secondary causes, simply reviewing these red flags can be vital in early diagnosis and management. If there is an underlying cause, the systemic or neurologic symptoms may show up more clearly over time.[14] In addition, when pain is refractory to traditional treatments, the diagnosis should always be reassessed.

TRIGEMINAL NEURALGIA

Neuralgias are characterized by paroxysmal, short-lasting lancinating pain at the distribution of the culprit nerve. Different neuralgias exist in the orofacial region, and they are summarized in **Table 1**.[18–21] In this article, the authors cover TN, the most common form of facial neuralgia.

Cause and Epidemiology

TN may develop without any apparent cause or secondary to another disorder. Although TN is the most common form of facial neuralgia, the prevalence is rare in the general population, with estimates of 5 to 12 cases per 100,000 people in the United States and with a slight female predilection.[18] Most commonly, TN affects those over the age of 50 years with the an incidence of 25.9 per 100,000 people per

Table 1
Orofacial neuralgias

Name	Nerve Involved	Pain Distribution	Triggers
Trigeminal neuralgia,[18–20] most common cranial neuralgia	• One or more divisions of the trigeminal nerve, which supplies the sensory innervation of the face and oral cavity • Usually unilateral, the right side is affected more often than the left	• Distributed along with the maxillary or mandibular division of the trigeminal nerve, affecting the cheek or chin on one side • Ophthalmic division only involvement is rare (<5%) • Some progress to more divisions of the trigeminal nerve over time	• Spontaneous or light touch on the skin, activities with movement of the face, jaw, or tongue, or a thermal stimulus • Most frequent trigger maneuvers are gentle touching of the face and talking[20,21] • Trigger zones are predominantly reported in the perioral and nasal region[21]
Glossopharyngeal neuralgia[18]	• Branches of the glossopharyngeal nerve • Innervate oropharynx, throat, the base of the tongue, tonsillar fossa, and tympanic plexus	• Unilateral deep stabbing pain of the throat • May radiate to the tongue, tonsil area, or the ear— • Occasionally accompanied by cardiovascular symptoms: bradycardia, asystole, hypotension, or syncope owing to crossover with vagus nerve (vago-glosso-pharyngeal neuralgia)	• Swallowing, chewing, talking, coughing, yawning, or turning the head • Some patients stop eating or drinking to avoid an attack
Nervus intermedius neuralgia (geniculate neuralgia)[18]	• Sensory branch of the facial nerve • Innervates the external auditory meatus, pinna of the ear, and some of the skin below the ear lobe	• Pain deep in the auditory canal of the ear, the external structures of the ear, the palate, tongue, or deeply in the facial musculature • Rarely, the anterior two-thirds of the tongue and soft palate involved • Can be associated with tearing, salivation, bitter taste, tinnitus, or vertigo on the unilateral side • Can be associated with herpes zoster	• Swallowing, talking, or stimulation of the ear canal

| Superior laryngeal neuralgia[18] | • A sensory branch of the vagus nerve
• Innervates the cricothyroid muscles and the vocal cords— | • Pain at the side of the thyroid cartilage, pyriform sinus, or angle of the jaw—
• May extend to the posterior auricular region, shoulder, upper thorax, or palate if auricular branch is also involved | • Talking, swallowing, yawning, coughing, turning the head, or straining the voice
• Sometimes an urge to swallow |
| Occipital and other branch neuralgia[18] | • Somatic sensory branches of the cervical spinal nerves | • Sudden, unilateral pains in the back of the head or neck | • Innocuous stimuli to the occipital region of the back of the head, neck, and shoulder muscles |

Data from Hupp WS, Firriolo FJ. Cranial neuralgias. Dent Clin North Am. 2013;57(3):481-95.[18]

year for patients over 80 years of age.[19] In a systematic review published in 2016, a higher prevalence of 0.03% to 0.3% was reported.[22]

Clinical Presentation

The recurrent sudden intense pain is limited to the distribution of one or more divisions of the trigeminal nerve. Pain triggered by innocuous stimuli is a key diagnostic feature of TN,[20,21] and it is reported by 91% to 99% of patients.[20] In addition, patients may report concomitant, continuous pain of moderate intensity within the affected divisions. Rarely, TN presents bilaterally.[19,20] Di Stefano and colleagues[21] studied triggering maneuvers in 140 patients with TN. The 2 most frequent triggers were (1) gentle touching of the face (79%) predominantly around the perioral and nasal region, and (2) talking (54%).[21] The trigger zones for TN can also be located intraorally along the distribution of second and third divisions of the trigeminal nerve.[20] Because of severe pain, patients usually refrain from touching the trigger area/zone or avoid performing triggering maneuvers.

Clinical Evaluation and Diagnosis

The initial diagnosis of TN is made clinically, using the patient's history to guide decision making. Clinical evaluation includes replicating and observing the patient's pain by triggers, mapping the trigger zone and the dermatome involvement.[20] Although most TN cases are classical, it is essential to rule out secondary TN. Neuroimaging with MRI is necessary for all patients with clinically established TN. Other investigations, such as neurophysiologic recording of trigeminal reflexes or trigeminal evoked potentials, are recommended for patients who cannot undergo MRI.

The International Classification of Orofacial Pain (ICOP) diagnostic criteria[23] define TN as recurrent paroxysms of unilateral facial pain in the distribution of one or more divisions of the trigeminal nerve, with no radiation beyond and fulfilling the following characteristics: lasting from a fraction of a second to 2 minutes, severe intensity, electric shocklike, shooting, stabbing, or sharp in quality, and precipitated by innocuous stimuli within the affected trigeminal distribution. The pain is not accounted for by another ICOP or International Classification of Headache Disorders (ICHD-3) diagnosis.

There are different classification systems, but, in general, TN can be categorized into classical, secondary, and idiopathic forms.[20,23,24]

(a) Classical TN is the most common form. The pain is caused by neurovascular compression of the trigeminal nerve root, causing atrophy or displacement of the nerve root, which can be verified by MRI or during a surgical procedure.[19,20,23,24]

In this classical form, there is a pain-free refractory period between the episodes, and it is termed classical TN, which is purely paroxysmal in the ICOP classification.[24] When there is a persistent background pain between attacks in the affected area, it is classified as "classical trigeminal neuralgia with concomitant continuous pain."[24] This type was formerly known as "atypical trigeminal neuralgia; trigeminal neuralgia type 2." The continuous background pain is from peripheral or central sensitization of the affected nerves.[23,24]

(b) Secondary TN or symptomatic TN is caused by an underlying pathologic condition. In ICOP classification,[24] secondary TN is further subcategorized by the attributing underlying diseases, such as TN attributed to multiple sclerosis, TN attributed to space-occupying lesions, and TN attributed to other causes. This accounts for up to 15% of cases of all TN,[20] and clinical examination shows sensory changes in a significant proportion of these patients.[23] Many of these patients also have continuous background pain with the triggering episodes.[19]

(c) Idiopathic TN is termed when there is no abnormality by electrophysiologic testing and by MRI. ICOP subclassified idiopathic TN into idiopathic TN, purely paroxysmal, and idiopathic TN with concomitant continuous pain, based on the presentation of pain.[24]

Management

Pharmacologic management with anticonvulsants is the first-line therapy for patients with TN.[19,20] Carbamazepine has been shown to be the most efficacious and is considered the gold standard in the treatment of TN. However, it has a high side-effect profile and possible serious complications, especially because of hepatic enzyme induction.[20] Oxcarbazepine is another first-line drug with a better side-effect profile than carbamazepine and similar efficacy.[19] These medications successfully control the TN pain attack in 70% to 90% of the patients regardless of the cause.[19,20,25] The second line of treatment includes baclofen and lamotrigine, and the third-line drugs are levetiracetam, topiramate, gabapentin, pregabalin, and local injection of onabotulinum toxin A at the trigger zones.[19] These second- and third-line medications are used in patients who cannot tolerate the first-line drugs as a stand-alone therapy or as add-on medications to reduce dosage (side effects) of the first-line drugs.

Surgical procedures are either invasive or destructive, and they are reserved for a patient with at least 3 failed pharmacologic therapies owing to their lack of effect or intolerable side effects. Microvascular decompression (MVD) is the most invasive yet the most effective permanent treatment of classical TN cases.[20,25] Percutaneous rhizotomy to the trigeminal ganglion or root using radiofrequency thermocoagulation, glycerol injection, or balloon compression is less invasive and is preferred when MRI does not demonstrate any nerve root compression.[25] Gamma-knife radiosurgery for TN is the more recently introduced treatment and is recommended for patients who cannot undergo MVD. Pain relief effect can take 6 to 8 weeks, and it has a ~50% recurrence of pain after 3 years.[19,20]

TRIGEMINAL NEUROPATHY (CONTINUOUS)
Posttraumatic Trigeminal Neuropathic Pain

Cause and epidemiology

By definition, PTTN is caused by a trauma to the sensory nerve, which results in a dysfunction of the nerve, causing pain and/or other sensory disturbance. Although it can affect anyone, it is more commonly reported in women of around 45 to 50 years old and who may also suffer from other chronic pain disorders. Patients with PTTN often see several providers and undergo multiple invasive, dental treatments, such as root canal treatment, apicectomy, or extraction, for the treatment of pain. None of these treatments improve the pain and may, on the other hand, exacerbate it. These procedures could potentially be the cause of PTTN. However, in many cases, pain exists preceding the invasive treatment, making the diagnosis difficult. The key feature for patients with PTTN is that the quality of the pain after the offending procedure is different from before. For example, severe pulsating pain aggravated by cold stimuli as seen in acute pulpitis, changing to mild to moderate dull continuous pain as seen in PTTN, after a root canal treatment indicates that the pain was from peripheral nerve damage.

The estimated prevalence of PTTN following major trauma is 3%.[26] This is similar to Nixdorf and colleagues,[27] who reported a prevalence of 3.4% of nonodontogenic pain after endodontic procedures.

Clinical presentation

The clinical presentation of PTTN widely varies, possibly because of the extent of the injury and neuroplastic change following the injury. The pain may be continuous, spontaneous, or evoked and accompanied by positive (dysesthesia, hyperalgesia, allodynia) or negative (numbness) neuronal symptoms. The patient may also complain of heat/cold or a swelling sensation. In addition, the patient commonly reports burning, dull, achy pain, or tingling pain, but a report of other characteristics of pain is also common, such as throbbing pain or a sharp paroxysmal pain.

Clinical evaluation and diagnosis

ICOP[22] defines this pain as follows:

(A) Pain, in a neuroanatomically plausible area within the distribution of one or both trigeminal nerves, persisting or recurring for greater than 3 months and fulfilling criteria C and D

(B) Both of the following
  1. History of a mechanical, thermal, radiation, or chemical injury to the peripheral trigeminal nerve
  2. Diagnostic test confirmation of a lesion of the peripheral trigeminal nerve explaining the pain

(C) Onset within 6 months after the injury

(D) Associated with somatosensory symptoms and/or signs in the same neuroanatomically plausible distribution

(E) Not better accounted for by another ICOP or ICHD-3 diagnosis. There are many previously used terms that may now fall under the diagnostic criteria of PTTN or PIFP. These previously used terms are painful PTTN, atypical facial pain, atypical odontalgia, persistent dentoalveolar pain, and phantom tooth pain. Clinicians are now discouraged from using these previous terms to share the consensus in diagnosing these conditions.

Although the "identifiable history of trauma" is one of the requirements for diagnosing PTTN, sometimes it is challenging to identify such an event. Diagnosis can be difficult because the exact degree of injury required to cause PTTN is may be unknown. For example, chronic infection, chronic ischemic injury, and minor trauma are argued to cause PTTN. In these cases, the evidence of trauma may not be obvious, making it more difficult to diagnose.

Diagnostic testing: anesthetic test for determining peripheral versus central neuropathy. Sometimes, patients may report pain in the area with no clinical evidence of inflammation, infection, or trauma. In these cases, doctors may think the pain originates from psychological problems. However, the patient may be experiencing PTTN and not psychological pain. Because neuropathic pain is derived from a dysfunction of a damaged nerve, if the damaged peripheral nerve can be blocked, the pain should be alleviated.

1. Have the patient scale their pain using the visual analogue scale (using 10-cm line) or numerical rating scale (from 0 to 10 or 0 to 100).
2. Apply topical anesthetic at the site of pain.
3. Ask the patient to rate the pain again after 3 and 6 minutes.
4. If the pain persists, consider local infiltration and rate the pain again after 3 and 6 minutes.
5. If the pain persists, consider nerve block to see if this will change their pain.

With central neuropathy, whereby neuroplastic change has occurred in the CNS, or psychological source of pain, an anesthetic test will not eliminate pain. This test can be useful to see if any additional dental treatment may be beneficial. For example, if a patient is reporting pain on a tooth and anesthetizing the area does not provide pain relief, then performing dental procedures would not be the recommended treatment. In fact, it could exacerbate the pain.

Management

PTTN can be managed with both topical and systemic medications. Topical medications include local anesthetic; compounded medications, including various neuroleptic and anesthetic medications; and capsaicin. These topical medications are then applied locally to the site of pain using a neurosensory stent, which would shield the affected tissues and contain the topical medication in place. If the topical medications are not effective, then systemic medications should be considered. These include the gabapentinoids (gabapentin, pregabalin, or mirogabalin), tricyclic antidepressants (amitriptyline, nortriptyline), serotonin-norepinephrine reuptake inhibitors (duloxetine), and tramadol.

Any additional, invasive procedures must be avoided, as they have a risk of exacerbating the patient's pain. Instead, referral to (1) an endodontist for ruling-out odontogenic pain, such as chronic periapical periodontitis or crack/fracture; or (2) an orofacial pain specialist for a further evaluation is strongly recommended when a patient reports pain without an obvious cause.

Trigeminal Postherpetic Neuralgia

Cause and epidemiology

Trigeminal postherpetic neuralgia is one form of PTTN, in which trauma to the nerve is caused by the varicella-zoster virus (VZV). Recurrent infection of VZV may damage the trigeminal nerve and result in continuous pain of the face, accompanied by positive (dysesthesia, hyperalgesia, allodynia) or negative (numbness) neuronal symptoms. Trigeminal postherpetic neuralgia of the face is most frequently seen on the first branch of the trigeminal nerve, rarely occurring in the patient younger than 40 years of age. The pain is often described as burning or tingling pain. It may be continuous and/or paroxysmal. In an immunocompromised patient, recurrent VZV infection is more common than in healthy individuals; clinical symptoms may be more atypical, and there may be more severe symptoms. This may lead to a higher development rate of trigeminal postherpetic neuralgia. A study done in South Korea reported the prevalence of herpes zoster and postherpetic neuralgia to be 18.54 and 2.88 per 1000 persons, respectively, and increased with deteriorating immune status.[28]

Clinical presentation

Usually, the pain occurs while the rash is still active, but, in some cases, the pain can develop later on, after the blisters have healed. In such cases, pale or light purple scars may be present as a sequela of the herpetic eruption. The critical part of the diagnosis is that there must be a history of herpes zoster infection.

Clinical evaluation and diagnosis

ICOP[22] defines this pain as follows:

(A) Unilateral facial pain in the distributions of a trigeminal nerve branch or nerve branches, persisting or recurring for greater than 3 months, and fulfilling criterion C
(B) Herpes zoster has affected the same trigeminal nerve branch or branches
(C) Pain developed in temporal relation to the acute herpes zoster infection
(D) Not better accounted for by another ICOP or ICHD-3 diagnosis

The anesthetic test described earlier may be able to alleviate the pain, aiding the diagnosis of peripheral sensitization.

Management

Management of trigeminal postherpetic neuralgia is similar to those of PTTN or any other neuropathic pain. Trigeminal postherpetic neuralgia responds well to topical or systemic treatment listed before, but there are some refractory cases that may significantly diminish the quality of life of the patient. Nerve block procedures, neural ablation, or onabotulinum toxin A injection are some other treatments for refractory cases. These procedures are discussed later in the trigeminal neuralgia section of this article.

Persistent Idiopathic Facial Pain

Cause and epidemiology

PIFP was previously called atypical facial pain.[29] If this occurred at a dental structure, then it was called atypical dental pain or atypical odontalgia.[30] ICOP now separates pain occurring in facial region and oral region in different diagnoses. However, these two are thought to share similar pathogenesis.

The exact pathophysiology of PIFP is yet unknown. However, some groups theorize that PIFP and PTTN may represent 2 extremes of a spectrum of clinical presentations, whereby PIFP is a disproportionate reaction to a mild injury.[29] According to ICOP diagnostic criteria written in later discussion, PIFP is suggestive of central sensitization (neuropathic pain involving central nervous system), as it is poorly localized and does not follow the distribution of a peripheral nerve. In contrast, PTTN involves more peripheral nerves, as the pain is distributed within a neuroanatomically plausible area of one or both trigeminal nerves.

The ambiguity of the condition and diagnostic criteria allow it to be easily confused with other chronic pain conditions, leading to misdiagnoses. This makes it difficult to estimate the prevalence and also to produce a consensus for a treatment strategy. Based on the best current knowledge, Mueller and colleagues[31] reported the estimated lifetime prevalence to be 0.03%. This pain is most commonly seen in women with a mean age of onset in their mid-40s.

Clinical presentation

The pain is poorly localized and does not follow the distribution of a peripheral nerve, and clinically, the neurologic examination is normal. In some cases, the pain is hard to replicate, and local infiltration of anesthetic may not eliminate pain.

Clinical evaluation and diagnosis

ICOP[24] defines PIFP as follows:

(A) Facial pain fulfilling criteria B and C
(B) Recurring daily for greater than 2 h/d for greater than 3 months
(C) Pain has both of the following characteristics:
    1. Poorly localized, and not following the distribution of a peripheral nerve
    2. Dull, aching, or nagging quality
(D) Clinical and radiographic examinations are normal, and local causes have been excluded
(E) Not better accounted for by another ICOP or ICHD-3 diagnosis

ICOP diagnostic criteria for persistent idiopathic dentoalveolar pain is the same as that for PIFP except that the pain is located intraorally in the dentoalveolar region.

Management

There is yet no consensus for the management of PIFP. Because this diagnosis may include diseases with different pathogenesis, one treatment may work for one patient but not for another. Some may involve pain in a wider region of the body; some may involve dysfunction of central inhibitory process, or some may only involve peripheral neuroplastic changes. Because patients with PIFP are known to have comorbid psychological conditions, a multidisciplinary approach is recommended.

Burning Mouth Syndrome

Cause and epidemiology
The general population prevalence of BMS varies from 0.1% to 3.9%.[32] BMS is broadly categorized into 2 types: primary and secondary. Secondary BMS is a whole group of diseases that can cause a burning sensation in the mouth. This includes local or systemic infection (eg, candidiasis), nutrition deficiencies (eg, vitamin B group, zinc, iron), systemic conditions (eg, iron deficiency anemia, pernicious anemia), an autoimmune disorder (eg, lichen planus), or side effects of medications taken for another disease (eg, antihypertensive medication).

Many pathogeneses of BMS are discussed, but none is definitive. BMS is thought to be caused by mutifactorial factors. The general consensus is that BMS involves neuropathic components and not only psychological elements, as it is commonly accompanied by neurologic dysfunction, like dysgeusia.

BMS is commonly seen in the female patient, with a marked male-to-female ratio of 1:8–9. It is prominent in perimenopausal to postmenopausal women and extremely rare in ages younger than 50 years.

Clinical presentations
A burning sensation of the oral mucosa is reported without obvious pathologic condition. The pain most commonly affects the anterior two-thirds of the tongue, especially in the tip of the tongue. It may affect labial mucosa and the anterior palate, but almost never involves the floor of the mouth. The burning pain is accompanied by xerostomia and dysgeusia. Patients report their pain is better when they are eating. Clinical examination reveals normal mucosa and normal salivary flow.

Clinical evaluation and diagnosis
When all causes of secondary BMS are excluded, and the patient is still reporting a burning sensation of the mouth, then primary BMS could be the endpoint of diagnosis. ICOP[22] defines this pain as follows:

A. Oral pain fulfilling criteria B and C
B. Recurring daily for greater than 2 h/d for greater than 3 months
C. Pain has both of the following characteristics:
　　1. Burning quality
　　2. Superficial feeling in the oral mucosa
D. Oral mucosa is of normal appearance, and local or systemic causes have been excluded
E. Not better accounted for by another ICOP or ICHD-3 diagnosis

Management
There are a few suggested treatments for BMS, but only 3 of these are shown to have some level of evidence in a Cochrane review[33]: topical clonazepam, cognitive behavioral therapy, and alpha-lipoic acid.

DISCUSSION

Dentists are well trained to detect oral pain originating from infections, inflammation, and trauma. However, detection and management of neuropathic or psychological pain are not well understood in general. Specific diagnosis and management can be referred to an orofacial pain specialist. However, these patients with neuropathic pain first visit general practitioners. It has been reported that more than 80% of patients with TN saw a dentist or dentists for pain, and two-thirds of those patients received invasive, unnecessary dental treatments.[33] Therefore, it is up to general dentists to recognize these conditions and be able to connect the patients to a specialist or specialists for further evaluation and treatment.

SUMMARY

Patients with unexplained orofacial pain need to be thoroughly assess by history taking and physical examination. Identifying red flags is essential for early diagnosis and management of neuropathic orofacial pain from the underlying cause, such as brain tumor or cancer.

CLINICS CARE POINTS

- General dentists may be the first providers to see patients with neuropathic pain.
- Thorough history taking is the crucial step in recognizing neuropathic orofacial pain.
- Neuropathic orofacial pain conditions must be recognized to avoid unnecessary dental treatment and to initiate proper referral and treatment.
- Reassess the diagnosis when the pain is refractory to standard dental treatment.

DISCLOSURE

The authors declare no commercial or financial conflicts of interest related to the contents of this article.

REFERENCES

1. Kohli D, Thomas DC. Orofacial pain: time to see beyond the teeth. J Am Dent Assoc 2020;S0002-8177(20):30418-9.
2. Crandall JA. An introduction to orofacial pain. Dent Clin North Am 2018;62(4):511-23.
3. International Association for the Study of Pain. IASP Taxonomy Working Group. Part III pain terms: a current list with definitions and notes on usage (Updated 2011) Available at: https://www.iasp-pain.org/wp-content/uploads/2021/07/Part_III-PainTerms.pdf. Accessed August 26, 2021.
4. Baron R, Binder A, Wasner G. Neuropathic pain: diagnosis, pathophysiological mechanisms, and treatment. Lancet Neurol 2010;9(8):807-19.
5. Benoliel R, Eliav E. Neuropathic orofacial pain. Oral Maxillofac Surg Clin N Am 2008;20(2):237-254, vii.
6. Christoforou J. Neuropathic orofacial pain. Dent Clin North Am 2018;62(4):565-84.
7. Renton T. Chronic pain and overview or differential diagnoses of non-odontogenic orofacial pain. Prim Dent J 2019;7(4):71-86.
8. Bender SD. Assessment of the orofacial pain patient. Dent Clin North Am 2018;62(4):525-32.
9. The American Academy of Orofacial Pain. Orofacial pain: guidelines for assessment, diagnosis, and management. Quintessence Publishing; 2018.
10. Dieb W, Moreau N, Chemla I, et al. Neuropathic pain in the orofacial region: the role of pain history. A retrospective study. J Stomatol Oral Maxillofac Surg 2017;118(3):147-50.

11. Sheeler RD, Garza I, Vargas BB, et al. Chronic daily headache: ten steps for primary care providers to regain control. Headache 2016;56(10):1675–84.
12. Sarlani E, Balciunas BA, Grace EG. Orofacial Pain–Part II: Assessment and management of vascular, neurovascular, idiopathic, secondary, and psychogenic causes. AACN Clin Issues 2005;16(3):347–58.
13. Kreiner M, Falace D, Michelis V, et al. Quality difference in craniofacial pain of cardiac vs. dental origin. J Dent Res 2010;89(9):965–9.
14. Moazzam AA, Habibian M. Patients appearing to dental professionals with orofacial pain arising from intracranial tumors: a literature review. Oral Surg Oral Med Oral Pathol Oral Radiol 2012;114(6):749–55.
15. Van Abel K, Starkman S, O'Reilly A, et al. Craniofacial pain secondary to occult head and neck tumors. Otolaryngology-Head Neck Res 2014;150(5):813–7.
16. Hwang WJ, Huang K, Huang JS. Amyotrophic lateral sclerosis presenting as the temporomandibular disorder: a case report and literature review. Cranio 2017; 28:1–5.
17. Aerden T, Grisar K, Neven P, et al. Numb chin syndrome as a sign of mandibular metastasis: a case report. Int J Surg Case Rep 2017;31:68–71.
18. Hupp WS, Firriolo FJ. Cranial neuralgias. Dent Clin North Am 2013;57(3):481–95.
19. Jones MR, Urits I, Ehrhardt KP, et al. A comprehensive review of trigeminal neuralgia. Curr Pain Headache Rep 2019;23(10):74.
20. Cruccu G, Di Stefano G, Truini A. Trigeminal neuralgia. N Engl J Med 2020;383(8): 754–62.
21. Di Stefano G, Maarbjerg S, Nurmikko T, et al. Triggering trigeminal neuralgia. Cephalalgia 2018;38(6):1049–56.
22. De Toledo IP, Conti Réus J, Fernandes M, et al. Prevalence of trigeminal neuralgia: a systematic review. J Am Dent Assoc 2016;147(7):570–6.e2.
23. International Classification of Orofacial Pain, 1st edition (ICOP). Cephalalgia 2020;40(2):129–221. Available at: https://journals.sagepub.com/doi/full/10.1177/0333102419893823. Accessed September 23, 2021.
24. Headache Classification Committee of the International Headache Society (IHS). The International Classification of Headache Disorders. 3rd edition 2013. Available at. https://ichd-3.org/13-painful-cranial-neuropathies-and-other-facial-pains/13-1-trigeminal-neuralgia/13-1-1-classical-trigeminal-neuralgia/. Accessed August 26, 2021.
25. Bendtsen L, Zakrzewska JM, Abbott J, et al. European Academy of Neurology guideline on trigeminal neuralgia. Eur J Neurol 2019;26(6):831–49.
26. Baad-Hansen L, Benoliel R. Neuropathic orofacial pain: facts and fiction. Cephalalgia 2017;37(7):670–9.
27. Nixdorf DR, Moana-Filho EJ, Law AS, et al. Frequency of non-odontogenic pain after endodontic therapy: a systematic review and meta-analysis. J Endod 2010;36(9):1494–8.
28. Cheong C, Lee TJ. Prevalence and healthcare utilization of herpes zoster and postherpetic neuralgia in South Korea: disparity among patients with different immune statuses. Epidemiol Health 2014;36:e2014012.
29. Benoliel R, Gaul C. Persistent idiopathic facial pain. Cephalalgia 2017;37(7): 680–91.
30. Baad-Hansen L, Pigg M, Ivanovic SE, et al. Intraoral somatosensory abnormalities in patients with atypical odontalgia–a controlled multicenter quantitative sensory testing study. Pain 2013;154(8):1287–94.

31. Mueller D, Obermann M, Yoon MS, et al. Prevalence of trigeminal neuralgia and persistent idiopathic facial pain: a population-based study. Cephalalgia 2011; 31(15):1542–8.

32. McMillan R, Forssell H, Buchanan JA, et al. Interventions for treating burning mouth syndrome. Cochrane Database Syst Rev 2016;11(11):CD002779.

33. von Eckardstein KL, Keil M, Rohde V. Unnecessary dental procedures as a consequence of trigeminal neuralgia. Neurosurg Rev 2015;38(2):355–60.

Oral Health Advocacy for People with Special Health Care Needs

Kimberly Marie Espinoza, DDS, MPH

KEYWORDS

- Advocacy • Cultural humility • Special care dentistry • Social determinants of health

KEY POINTS

- Oral health care providers can engage in critical self-reflection as a starting point for developing cultural humility in the care of people with disabilities.
- Power imbalances between health care providers and patients with disabilities can be addressed using collaborative approaches that support autonomy, and by addressing power imbalances based on ableism hierarchies.
- Cultural humility also includes advocating to improve the social determinants of health that contribute to health inequities, including access to quality health care, economic stability and educational attainment, and social and environmental contexts.

Abbreviations	
PSHCNs	people with special healthcare needs
CSHCNs	children with special healthcare needs
SDH	social determinants of health
ADLs	activities of daily living

INTRODUCTION

Advocacy work within the field of Special Care Dentistry is needed to help reduce oral health inequities for people with special health care needs (PSHCNs). This population has high rates of untreated dental decay and periodontal disease, as well as more difficulty accessing dental care.[1–3] Disabled individuals also report more difficulty finding care that meets their needs, including care that is culturally appropriate.[4]

By definition, Special Care Dentistry entails oral health care for "people with physical, medical, developmental, or cognitive conditions which limit their ability to receive routine dental care"[5] (**Box 1**). When referencing limitations to routine dental care, a medical model of disability would have the clinician focusing on the impairments of

Department of Oral Medicine, University of Washington, School of Dentistry, Box 356370, Seattle, WA 98195-6370, USA
E-mail address: kmespino@uw.edu

Dent Clin N Am 66 (2022) 245–259
https://doi.org/10.1016/j.cden.2022.01.004
dental.theclinics.com

Box 1
Defining special care dentistry populations

People with special health care needs (PSHCNs): People "who have or are at increased risk for chronic physical, developmental, behavioral or emotional conditions and also require health and related services of a type or amount beyond that required by [individuals] generally." A special health care need (SHCN) may or may not lead to a disability.[7]

People with disability: The World Health Organization defines disability as impairments of body functions and structures, activity limitations, and participation restrictions that result from interactions between health conditions, personal factors, and environmental factors. A person with a disability may have special health care needs, but an association is not always present.[8]

Special care dentistry population: Special Care Dentistry involves care for "people with physical, medical, developmental, or cognitive conditions which limit their ability to receive routine dental care." People with special health care needs, as with disabled individuals, are more likely to have limitations in their ability to receive routine dental care. However, not all individuals with special health care needs and/or disability will experience such limitations.[5]

---

individuals with disability. In advocating for PSHCNs, a change in focus is indicated. The social model of disability posits that limitations are created by the environment.[6] This article reviews the environmental limitations to oral health often encountered by these populations. Furthermore, the article outlines advocacy pathways for the oral health professional with a cultural humility focus.

Developing cultural humility in the care of patients with disability is a good start in efforts to advocate for this population's oral health. Cultural humility in health care is characterized by the following 4 main concepts[9]:

1. Critical self-reflection
2. Addressing power imbalances in health care relationships
3. Advocacy for change to improve the social determinants of health (SDH)
4. A lifelong process of ongoing learning and action

This article explores these concepts and gives the oral health professional related recommendations for disability advocacy.

CRITICAL SELF-REFLECTION

Critical self-reflection is a process by which individuals become more self-aware. This is done through analysis of one's own assumptions about self, including one's own identities, experiences, skills, beliefs, actions, and biases.[9,10] For example, a health care provider engaging in critical self-reflection might humbly consider what they know versus what they do not know when it comes to the experiences of patients with disability. A provider might also consider their own relationship and experiences with disability and how their beliefs and experiences might enhance or limit their ability to take the perspectives of their disabled patients.

Critical self-reflection also involves an examination of how one is influenced by interpersonal, situational, and societal contexts.[10] For example, a provider might examine how their beliefs and actions related to disability are influenced by the larger context of an ableist society, or the smaller contexts of the health care setting in which they work, or specific individual interactions.

Self-critique, another element of critical self-reflection, involves examining those areas where the provider might seek transformation.[10] For example, a provider might recognize an area where one needs more education related to a disability concept, such as the social model of disability. Another example would be recognizing when a change in one's course of action or way of thinking is indicated, such as to avoid unintentionally stigmatizing language. Although it is important to practice self-critique in developing cultural humility, these skills will be counterproductive if self-critique is overdone and prevents the individual from achieving their transformative goals. Having a growth mindset in this area, knowing that cultural humility can be improved with learning and practice, will aid the practitioner in engaging in critical self-reflection and self-critique in a productive way.[11]

CLINICS ADVOCACY POINTS

- Engage in critical self-reflection related to knowledge about disability, experience with disability, and potential biases related to disability.
- Assess clinical skills, including skills in patient communication and facilitation techniques for supporting patients with disability.
- Assess the state of the dental practice in terms of accessibility and ability to deliver meaningful care to disabled individuals.
- Seek resources for education without imposing on individual disabled individuals. Examples include content published by disabled people, classes on disability studies, continuing education courses, and research articles.
- Maintain a growth mindset and seek solutions to gaps in accessibility, skills, comfort, and knowledge.

ADDRESSING POWER IMBALANCES

Power imbalances in health care relationships occur on multiple levels. Two significant types of power imbalances are those which are positional in nature as well as those associated with social identity groups.

Positional Power Imbalances

Positional power imbalances involve power differentials in positions of authority, where one individual holds more power over another, owing to the setting and nature of their position.[9] Examples of power imbalances in this area include those between employer and employee, between dentist and dental assistant, and between provider and patient. Addressing these power imbalances requires the person in the position of authority to moderate appropriate use of their power. Health care providers typically hold great influence over patients during the course of their care. The health care provider is the expert in their field and decides which care options to present to the patient. Similarly, the dental team should recognize that the patient is the expert in their own experiences, values, and needs.

Fully ascertaining the patient's area of expertise, and understanding their treatment wishes, is more challenging in certain situations. For example, when there are impairments in expressive or receptive communication, more attention is required in supporting communication needs. For some individuals, such as those with advanced dementia or significant intellectual disability, decision making may be delegated to a surrogate decision maker, such as a legal guardian. In these cases, the health care team should work to determine how best to support patient autonomy within this context. Additional discussion of informed consent for patients with disability is given in **Box 2**.

Box 2
Considerations in obtaining informed consent for patients with disabilities

Presumed competence: Providers should assume that disabled individuals can make their own decisions.

Legal competency to consent: People who have been assigned a legal guardian for medical decision making no longer have the legal right to make their own health care decisions. This is determined by the court system. Guardianship is restrictive because it takes away the rights of the person with a disability and gives these rights to someone else (a legal guardian).[12] Guardianship is meant to be limited to cases where there is no safe alternative.

Decision-making capacity: Capacity relates to whether an individual has the ability to understand their health care conditions, and the risks, benefits, and alternatives to care. To give consent that is truly informed, an individual must not only understand what's at stake but also appreciate how these stakes affect them personally, and reason through the options to come to a decision.[13] Decision-making capacity is procedure specific. For example, an individual may have the capacity to consent to dental prophylaxis, but not to general anesthesia. Decision-making capacity cannot be based on diagnosis alone, nor provider perceptions about the quality of choices patients make.

Discrepancies between competency and capacity: The terms competency and capacity are often used interchangeably; however, it is important to be able to differentiate between these concepts, regardless of the terminology used. Discrepancies between capacity and competency can create legal and ethical dilemmas. One example is if a patient legally can make their own decisions but does not have the capacity to understand the proposed treatment in order to give informed consent. Supported decision making may be needed in these cases.

Assent to care: Minors, as well as adults with a legal guardian, are generally not able to provide informed consent for health care procedures. Providers should assess if the individual in such a situation assents, or agrees, to the proposed care. Ethical dilemmas can present when consent is given from a parent or guardian, but assent is not given from the patient.

Supported decision making: Supported decision making focuses on supporting patients in understanding and considering their treatment options in order to make their own decisions. This can be as simple as talking to a friend about one's health care options, or more coordinated, such as creating a supported decision-making agreement between the individual wanting support and the person they have chosen to support them. Advocacy groups are calling for more access to supported decision making for disabled individuals in order to avoid more restrictive alternatives, such as guardianship.[14]

Using techniques designed to support autonomy during patient-provider communication can also help address positional power imbalances. Three such techniques are reviewed here:

- *Person-centered interviewing* is an interviewing model that assures patient comfort and readiness for care, elicits all of the concerns a patient would like to discuss, and elicits the patient's symptom story, including the personal and emotional contexts, before moving on to provider-centric questions.[15]
- *Shared decision-making* is a collaborative decision-making model between provider and patient. Providers elicit and support patients' goals, preferences, and values and work together with patients to support their engagement in the decision-making process.[16]
- *Motivational interviewing* is a technique for supporting patient behavior change, founded on the spirit of collaboration, autonomy, and evocation.[17] Providers support patients where they are, in terms of their readiness to change, and help patients elicit their own solutions for moving toward desired behavior change.

Beyond the need to support patient autonomy during patient-provider discussions, dentistry is procedural in nature. Patients are vulnerable to whether the practitioner attends to their needs throughout each encounter. Patients are also vulnerable because of the closeness of dentistry to sensitive areas. Tolerating touch to the head and neck, including inside the mouth, is difficult for many. Tolerating water from dental handpieces, ultrasonic scalers, or the air-water syringe is another common challenge. This is especially true for individuals with oropharyngeal dysphagia or oral sensitivities, which are commonly experienced by people with developmental or neurologic disabilities.[18,19] Attention to the needs of patients, including their verbal and nonverbal cues during procedures, can affect power dynamics in the patient-provider relationship.

CLINICS ADVOCACY POINTS

- Practice active listening and a collaborative style in patient interactions, recognizing the patient's own areas of expertise.
- Presume competence for patients with disabilities and learn more about surrogate decision making and supported decision making for people who have difficulty understanding their health conditions and treatment options.
- Use interviewing techniques designed to promote patient autonomy, such as person-centered interviewing, shared decision making, and motivational interviewing.
- Find ways to assure comfort and give power back to patients during clinical care, such as seeking assent for procedures, giving breaks during treatment, and seeking alternatives to enhance patient comfort.

Social Identity Group Power Imbalances

The next category of power imbalances are those related to social identity groups. The ADDRESSING Influences framework, from the field of psychology, identifies a list of social identity groups where power imbalances are common in society, including in health care interactions.[20] These include the following:

- Age and generational influences
- Developmental disability
- Disability acquired later in life
- Religion and spiritual orientation
- Ethnicity and race
- Socioeconomic status
- Sexual orientation
- Indigenous heritage
- National origin
- Gender and gender identity

Inequities and systems of oppression

Social group power imbalances are tied to health inequities, which are unjust differences in health outcomes between populations.[21] Systems of oppression contribute to inequities via power hierarchies where one group of people have dominant status in society and another group of people have nondominant status in society. *Ableism*, for example, is the system of oppression that maintains power imbalances between disabled individuals and those without disabilities.[22] This does not imply that disabled people cannot experience empowerment or success, but that they are more likely to experience societal barriers, and more risk to their health, on the basis of their ability status than their nondisabled peers.

Within each element of the ADDRESSING Influences there is not always a clear-cut binary. Disabled individuals may experience marginalization differently based on personal and environmental factors, as well as the functional impact of their condition. In addition, the experience of marginalization may vary depending on whether the disability is more visible or less visible, and how their experience of disability interacts with their other identities.[20,23]

Ableism and society

Ableism, as with other systems of oppression, occurs on multiple interacting levels.[22] At the societal level, ableism includes those laws, societal norms, and structural factors, such as the health care system, which disadvantage disabled people. An example at this level would be a health care insurance system largely based on employment, when disabled individuals are more likely to be unemployed or underemployed.

Ableism and organizations

At the institutional level, ableism includes organizational practices and norms that disadvantage disabled people. In terms of oral health, policies related to dental school accreditation, dental school curricula, dental practice, and the culture of the dental profession may have the unintentional outcome of disadvantage to disabled people. An example might include past predoctoral accreditation standards, which until 2020, only required graduates to be competent in assesssing the needs of PSHCNs as opposed to managing their care.[24]

Ableism at the Individual Level

At the individual level, ableism includes individual beliefs, attitudes, and behaviors that harm disabled people. An example is thinking disabled people are inferior to nondisabled people, which results in discrimination. Although ableism can be intentional, much of what sustains these systems of oppression is unintentional.[22] An example of an unintentional interaction is assuming a disabled person must be treated in a special care dentistry clinic simply because of their disability. This can have the negative effect of inappropriately segregating disabled individuals from people without disability. Although some individuals with disability may benefit from the advanced services offered in a special care dentistry clinic, referral should be an individualized assessment and not based on diagnosis alone.

CLINICS ADVOCACY POINTS

- Actively seek ways to include disabled individuals into the dental practice; if there are very few patients with disabilities in the practice, actively address accessibility barriers and promote access.
- Address ways that ableism may manifest in the clinic setting, such as via unconscious biases from providers and staff.
- Train the entire health care team on appropriate disability language, including the nuances of person-first (e.g. "person with a disability" / "person with an intellectual disability") and identity-first (e.g. "disabled person" / "autistic person") language, and how to avoid ableist language, both spoken and in the health care record.[25]

- Avoid segregating disabled individuals into special care dentistry clinics or special hours within a practice; assess each individual's needs before considering referral and attempt to integrate care as much as possible.

ADVOCACY FOR CHANGE

The concept of cultural humility extends beyond self-work and addressing power imbalances in practice. It also includes advocacy for improving the SDH, which are environmental factors that affect health beyond the individual level.[26] The following are examples of SDH:

- Health care access and quality
- Economic stability
- Education access and quality
- Neighborhood and built environment
- Social and community context

Health Care Access and Quality

Health care access

Limited access to oral health care is a common concern among PSHCNs. For children with special health care needs (CSHCNs), dental care is the number one unmet need.[27,28] Adults similarly face difficulty accessing dental care.[2] This problem is multifactorial. Some of the reasons for limited access to oral health care are difficulty finding a dentist willing to treat, limited training for oral health professionals, and financial barriers.

Willingness to treat. Parents of CSHCNs report it is often difficult to find a dentist willing to treat their child.[29] Many People SHCNs have to travel long distances to find care, not being able to find care within the community in which they live.[30] Dentists are often hesitant to treat this population and concerned about their level of training and their staff level of training in treating PSHCNs.[31] Other causes of dentist hesitancy include perceived complexity of care, fear of emergencies, and financial concerns.[31]

Training and education. Dentists have historically felt ill prepared to treat PSHCNs. Hands-on training has been limited in many areas of special care dentistry, particularly in the care of patients with developmental disabilities.[31] The Commission on Dental Accreditation (CODA) enacted standards in 2004 that required dental graduates to be able to "*assess* the needs of patients with special needs," but did not include a requirement for competency in *treating* this population. Unfortunately, dental school administrators often feel pressures of a cramped curricula, which may contribute to educational deficiencies in this area. In one study, 50% of dental school deans reported the care of patients with special needs not to be a high priority in the curriculum.[32] In another study, less than 60% of administrators thought their dental schools were fully in compliance with the CODA standard, and 80% thought the school should spend more time teaching in this area.[33] In 2020, the CODA standard was enhanced to include *managing* the care of patients with special needs.[24] The aim is that future dental school graduates will have more training with these vulnerable populations and be more likely to provide treatment to these populations beyond graduation.

Similarly, opportunities for advanced training in the care of PSHCNs are limited. Although pediatric dentistry programs provide training in the management of CSHCNs, accreditation pathways for advanced education in adult special care dentistry and geriatric dentistry have not yet been developed.[34] Although residencies in general practice dentistry hold promise for advanced training in some areas of special care dentistry, training in this area is not consistent across programs.

Financial barriers. Health care access is also influenced by the cost of health care and how health care is financed. Disabled individuals have higher rates of work-related disability and are more likely to be unemployed or underemployed.[35] This results in this population having less access to work-funded health insurance, including dental insurance. Medicaid eligibility is high in this population. Among CSHCNs, 47% are Medicaid recipients, and among nonelderly adults with disabilities, 30% are Medicaid recipients.[36,37] The proportion of adults with developmental disabilities with Medicaid coverage is even higher.

Although states are mandated to include children's dental care under Medicaid, there is no such stipulation for adults. Coverage varies by states; Medicaid reimbursement rates are often low, and many providers opt not to enroll in the Medicaid program.[38] The result is that it is often difficult for Medicaid recipients to locate Medicaid providers for adult dental care services.

Health care quality

Another SDH is health care quality. Health care quality is defined by care that is not only equitable but also timely, efficient, person-centered, safe, and effective.[39]

Timely and efficient care. Delays in dental care can result in increased burden of disease, risk for complications, increased pain, and decreased quality of life. Compared to people without disability, individuals with limitations in physical functioning, cognitive limitations, and difficulty seeing or hearing are more likely to experience delays in care.[40] Delays in care are also more common among people who receive assistance with activities of daily living (ADLs), among people who receive assistance with instrumental ADLs, or those who experience participation restrictions, such as restrictions in ability to work or participate in social activities.[40]

Difficulty finding a dentist, long waiting lists, and the concentration of special care dentistry programs in urban areas all contribute to treatment delays. Many PSHCNs travel hours to receive dental care.[30] Long waiting lists for general anesthesia services are a common problem. Children with active dental pain who need care under general anesthesia typically wait almost a month for care.[41] Access to general anesthesia services for adults may be even more limited.[30,42] Barriers to general anesthesia services include limited access to hospital operating room block time for dentists, lower hospital reimbursement for dental procedures compared with medical procedures, and disruptions to the health care system attributable to COVID-19.[43] Treatment delays can also result from onerous processes for preauthorization approvals, justifications of medical necessity, and the limited numbers of hospital dentistry programs and providers.[43]

Beyond treatment delays, care efficiency is affected by the preparation of dental practices to meet the needs of their PSHCNs, who are more likely to need procedures rescheduled, need longer appointments, or have procedures completed over multiple visits. Practices need to be responsive to both the expected and the emerging needs experienced by PSHCNs during dental care.

Person-centered care. A key area of health care quality is person-centered care, which is care that "defines success not just by the resolution of clinical symptoms but also by whether patients achieve their desired outcomes."[44] This includes care that respects patient values, preferences, and needs, including emotional needs and physical comfort. Person-centered care also includes care that meets patient expectations regarding coordination of care and ease of navigation of the healthcare system.

One area of person-centered care that is particularly relevant for many disabled individuals is the assurance of needs related to autonomy. Disabled individuals often experience stigma from health care providers who make assumptions about the individual's ability to make their own decisions.[45] In addition, disabled individuals often report not feeling listened to by their provider, especially when communicating their own expectations and needs regarding the delivery of care.[45,46]

Another component of person-centered care for disabled individuals includes appropriate involvement of family members and caregivers. Disabled individuals often report that health care providers inappropriately defer to their family members or caregivers when discussing treatment options or plans of care, essentially "talking over" the individual with disability. Disabled individuals involve family members and caregivers in their care for different reasons, and the role of the family member or caregiver will vary depending on the individual patient's needs and preferences.

Safe and effective care. Safe and effective care is an essential component of quality in health care. People want care not only that is going to have good outcomes but also that will be done safely. Unfortunately, people with disabilities often report receiving care that is unsafe. For example, there are numerous reports of disabled patients being injured during transfers, such as from a wheelchair to another surface, or when the healthcare provider did not listen to their instructions.[46]

In addition to safety issues, care that is ineffective is also problematic. Effective care is defined as care that is evidence based and appropriately matched to patient need.[39] What constitutes effective care, including preventive care, interventions, and care facilitation techniques, is not always clear.[47] Unfortunately, the lack of effective care contributes to the oral health inequities for disabled individuals. As noted by the National Council on Disability, "…a lack of understanding of disability issues among health professionals can minimize the effectiveness of the services provided, thus creating another roadblock for those claiming their health care rights."[48]

Economic Stability and Educational Access/Quality

Disabled individuals are more likely to experience low income and have less access to employment.[35] Economic instability is one area that adversely affects health. It does this directly via limited access to pay for health care services, as well as indirectly, such as affecting educational opportunities.

Inequities persist in educational attainment for disabled individuals. For example, people with physical and cognitive disabilities report lower educational attainment than people without physical or cognitive disabilities.[49] There are numerous pathways by which educational attainment can affect health outcomes. A major pathway is economic, including higher paying and more stable jobs, more income, and more resources, such as employer-sponsored insurance, that can support health and access to health care.[50] Educational attainment is also tied to health behaviors, health literacy, stress levels, coping skills, and available social supports.[50]

In addition, education impacts health via the environments in which one lives. For example, the relationship between low educational attainment and disability varies significantly between states.[51] Reasons proposed for these interstate differences include variations in safety net resources for people with lower income, and contextual characteristics, such as the concentration of poverty, transportation systems, and the accessibility of the built environment.[51]

Neighborhood, Built Environment, and Social/Community Context

Health is strongly tied to the environments within which one lives, varying not only by ZIP code, but also even down to the census tract level.[52,53] In addition, the built environment has significant impact on disabled individuals. For example, lack of accessible sidewalks, wheelchair ramps, and elevators can limit the ability of people with a mobility disability to access community resources and move about safely in their communities. Similarly, small operatories in dental clinics, tight spaces for obtaining radiographs, and narrow hallways can contribute to access barriers. Although the Americans with Disabilities Act mandates certain accessibility features in places of public accommodation, including dental offices, many dental offices still remain inaccessible.[48]

Another factor affecting the environments within which disabled individuals live, particularly those with developmental disabilities, is congregate living arrangements. Historically, people with developmental disabilities often lived in large institutions, and some still live in such institutions today. Concerns about segregation, quality of life, and abuse and neglect led to the nationwide process of deinstitutionalization, where most of such institutions have closed, moving their residents into community settings. Although institutional settings often had access to dental care with a dentist on site at the facility, the dental community was generally ill prepared for the closing of these institutions, furthering have a big impact on health for those void in access to dental care.[54]

Today, many adults with developmental disabilities live in smaller group settings, such as adult family homes, with the support of paid caregivers. Other people with developmental disabilities live independently, or with family members and friends. The availability and quality of caregiving support can have a big impact on health for those needing such services. Caregivers can help people perform oral hygiene care at home, drive individuals to appointments, schedule appointments, and advocate for their loved ones within the healthcare system. Family members and caregivers can be a great resource and part of the healthcare team. Unfortunately, people with developmental disabilities experience high rates of abuse and neglect, often from trusted individuals.[55] This betrayal of trust not only directly impacts health via the harm that it causes but also indirectly impacts health through a history of trauma that affects one's ability to trust those in positions of power, such as health care providers.[56]

Finally, dental providers and their practices make up part of the local social and community context. Whether people are able to access care in the communities in which they live and whether they have good relationships with their health care providers have important impacts on health.

CLINICS ADVOCACY POINTS

- Advocate within the culture of dentistry to promote care for disabled individuals.
- Promote programs and policies that enhance access to care, such as enhanced general anesthesia care, Medicaid reform, and provider loan repayment programs.
- Promote enhanced reimbursement programs for populations particularly vulnerable to access barriers, such as for individuals with intellectual and developmental disabilities.
- Promote education in special care dentistry, including supporting educational institutions, strong educational standards, and the creation of advanced education programs.

- Prepare for the need for increased services in the community in areas where state institutions for people with developmental disabilities are still active and at risk of closure.
- Assess for signs of abuse and neglect and deliver trauma-informed care.
- Follow the lead of disability organizations who are working to improve the social determinants of health for disabled individuals.

LIFELONG PROCESS OF ONGOING LEARNING AND ACTION

The term cultural humility is used as an alternative to the term cultural competence.[9] "Competence" problematically implies that one can become a cultural expert, including expertise in cultures that are not one's own. Cultural humility rejects this notion and instead focuses on the humble nature of recognizing one's own limitations and areas needed for growth in the vast context of human diversity. Cultural humility in healthcare involves continually exploring what one knows and does not know, striving to do better, and seeking solutions for the stubborn and unjust nature of health inequities.[9]

DISCUSSION

The access to care barriers and oral health inequities faced by PSHCNs can seem insurmountable. However, there are always ways that healthcare providers can serve as advocates. Reducing oral health inequities requires a multipronged approach. Advocacy efforts can be particularly effective within the areas where one has the most influence, such as one's own dental practices and communities. In addition, effective advocacy efforts can be sought by partnering with community organizations already engaged in this work.[9] Advocacy efforts are most likely to be effective when they are nonpaternalistic and are responsive to the expressed needs of the communities served, particularly the individuals who experience the inequities themselves.[9,57]

SUMMARY

Special Care Dentistry focuses on oral healthcare for people with limitations to receiving routine dental care. These limitations are largely created by an environment that does not sufficiently meet the needs of these populations. Advocacy work within the field of Special Care Dentistry can help address these inequities and includes critical self-reflection, addressing both positional and social group power imbalances in healthcare, and advocacy for change to improve the SDH. Finally, developing cultural humility in this area requires a lifelong commitment to learning and action.

DISCLOSURE

The author has nothing to disclose.

REFERENCES

1. Ward LM, Cooper SA, Hughes-McCormack L, et al. Oral health of adults with intellectual disabilities: a systematic review. J Intellect Disabil Res 2019;63(11): 1359–78.
2. Rouleau T, Harrington A, Brennan M, et al. Receipt of dental care and barriers encountered by persons with disabilities. Spec Care Dentist 2011;31(2):63–7.

3. Kisely S, Baghaie H, Lalloo R, et al. A systematic review and meta-analysis of the association between poor oral health and severe mental illness. Psychosom Med 2015;77(1):83–92.

4. Miller SR. A qualitative study of the perspectives of individuals with disabilities about their health care experiences: implications for culturally appropriate health care. J Natl Med Assoc 2012;104(7–8):360–5.

5. SCDA. SCDA definitions. Available at: https://www.scdaonline.org/general/custom.asp?page=SCDADefinitions. Accessed September 27, 2021.

6. Thomas C. Rescuing a social relational understanding of disability. Scand J Disabil Res 2004;6(1):22–36.

7. Health Resources and Services Administration. Children and youth with special health care needs. 2020. Available at: https://mchb.hrsa.gov/maternal-child-health-topics/children-and-youth-special-health-needs. Accessed September 27, 2021.

8. World Health Organization. Towards a common language for functioning disability and health ICF. 2002. Available at: https://www.who.int/classifications/icf/icfbeginnersguide.pdf. Accessed September 27, 2021.

9. Tervalon M, Murray-García J. Cultural humility versus cultural competence: a critical distinction in defining physician training outcomes in multicultural education. J Health Care Poor Underserved 1998;9(2):117–25.

10. Smith E. Teaching critical reflection. Teach Higher Education 2011;16:211–23. https://doi.org/10.1080/13562517.2010.515022.

11. Lee RER. What's missing from the conversation: the growth mindset in cultural competency. 2015. Available at: https://www.nais.org/learn/independent-ideas/august-2015/what%E2%80%99s-missing-from-the-conversation-the-growth-m/. Accessed September 27, 2021.

12. Disability Rights Washington. How to avoid guardianship pitfalls. 2017. Available at: https://www.disabilityrightswa.org/publications/how-avoid-guardianship-pitfalls/. Accessed September 27, 2021.

13. Dastidar JG, Odden A. How do I determine if my patient has decision-making capacity? The Hospitalist 2011;8.

14. The Arc. Position statement on autonomy, decision-making supports, and guardianship. 2016. Available at: https://thearc.org/position-statements/autonomy-decision-making-supports-guardianship/. Accessed September 27, 2021.

15. The beginning of the interview: patient-centered interviewing. In: Fortin AHVI, Dwamena FC, Frankel RM, et al, editors. Smith's patient-centered interviewing: an evidence-based method. 4th edition. McGraw-Hill Education; 2019.

16. Agency for Healthcare Research and Quality. The CAHPS Ambulatory Care Improvement Guide. Practical strategies for improving patient experience. Section 6: strategies for improving patient experience with ambulatory care. 2017. Available at: https://www.ahrq.gov/sites/default/files/wysiwyg/cahps/quality-improvement/improvement-guide/6-strategies-for-improving/communication/cahps-strategy-section-6-i.pdf. Accessed September 27, 2021.

17. Moyers TB. The relationship in motivational interviewing. Psychotherapy (Chic) 2014;51(3):358–63.

18. Robertson J, Chadwick D, Baines S, et al. Prevalence of dysphagia in people with intellectual disability: a systematic review. Intellect Dev Disabil 2017;55(6):377–91.

19. Takizawa C, Gemmell E, Kenworthy J, et al. A systematic review of the prevalence of oropharyngeal dysphagia in stroke, Parkinson's disease, Alzheimer's disease, head injury, and pneumonia. Dysphagia 2016;31(3):434–41.

20. Hays PA. The new reality: diversity and complexity. In: Addressing cultural Complexities in practice: assessment, diagnosis, and Therapy. 3rd edition. American Psychological Association; 2016. p. 3–18. Available at: http://www.jstor.org/stable/j.ctv1chs0x7.4.

21. The root causes of health inequity. In: Baciu A, Negussie Y, Geller A, et al, editors. Communities in action: pathways to health equity. Washington (DC): National Academies Press. January; 2017.

22. Ostiguy B, Peters ML, Shlasko D. Ableism. In: Adams M, Bell LA, editors. Teaching for diversity and social justice. Routledge; 2016.

23. Davis NA. Invisible disability. Ethics 2005;116(1):153–213. https://doi.org/10.1086/453151. Available at:.

24. Garvin J. Predoctoral programs now required to educate students on managing patients with disabilities. ADA news. 2019. Available at: https://www.ada.org/en/publications/ada-news/2019-archive/october/predoctoral-programs-now-required-to-educate-students-on-managing-patients-with-disabilities. Accessed September 27, 2021.

25. Dunn DS, Andrews EE. Person-first and identity-first language: developing psychologists' cultural competence using disability language. Am Psychol 2015;70(3):255–64.

26. Office of Disease Prevention and Health Promotion. Social determinants of health. Available at: https://health.gov/healthypeople/objectives-and-data/social-determinants-health. Accessed September 27, 2021.

27. Nelson LP, Getzin A, Graham D, et al. Unmet dental needs and barriers to care for children with significant special health care needs. Pediatr Dent 2011;33(1):29–36.

28. Chi DL. Oral health for US children with special health care needs. Pediatr Clin North Am 2018;65(5):981–93.

29. Al Agili DE, Roseman J, Pass MA, et al. Access to dental care in Alabama for children with special needs: parents' perspectives. J Am Dent Assoc 2004;135(4):490–5.

30. ASTDD. Best practice approaches for state and community oral health programs. 2021. Available at: https://www.astdd.org/bestpractices-bpa-special-needs.pdf. Accessed September 27, 2021.

31. Casamassimo PS, Seale NS, Ruehs K. General dentists' perceptions of educational and treatment issues affecting access to care for children with special health care needs. J Dent Educ 2004;68(1):23–8.

32. Holder M, Waldman HB, Hood H. Preparing health professionals to provide care to individuals with disabilities. Int J Oral Sci 2009;1(2):66–71.

33. Clemetson JC, Jones DL, Lacy ES, et al. Preparing dental students to treat patients with special needs: changes in predoctoral education after the revised accreditation standard. J Dent Educ 2012;76(11):1457–65.

34. Hicks J, Vishwanat L, Perry M, et al. SCDA Task Force on a special care dentistry residency. Spec Care Dentist 2016;36(4):201–12.

35. Poverty, employment and disability: the next great civil rights battle. Alexander W. Hum Rights 2014;40(3):18–22.

36. Musumeci MB, Chidambaram P, Kaiser Family Foundation. Medicaid's role for children with special health care needs: a look at eligibility, services, and spending. 2019. Available at: https://www.kff.org/medicaid/issue-brief/medicaids-role-for-children-with-special-health-care-needs-a-look-at-eligibility-services-and-spending/. Accessed September 27, 2021.

37. Musumeci MB, Foutz J, Kaiser Family Foundation. Medicaid restructuring under the American Health Care Act and nonelderly adults with disabilities. 2017. Available at: https://www.kff.org/medicaid/issue-brief/medicaid-restructuring-under-the-american-health-care-act-and-nonelderly-adults-with-disabilities/. Accessed September 27, 2021.
38. Center for Health Care Strategies. Medicaid adult dental benefits coverage by state. 2019. Available at: https://www.chcs.org/media/Medicaid-Adult-Dental-Benefits-Overview-Appendix_091519.pdf. Accessed September 27, 2021.
39. Institute of Medicine (US). Committee on Quality of Health Care in America. Improving the 21st-century health care system. In: Crossing the quality chasm: a New health system for the 21st century. Washington (DC): National Academies Press (US); 2001.
40. Horner-Johnson W, Dobbertin K. Dental insurance and dental care among working-age adults: differences by type and complexity of disability. J Public Health Dent 2016;76(4):330–9.
41. Lewis CW, Nowak AJ. Stretching the safety net too far waiting times for dental treatment. Pediatr Dent 2002;24(1):6–10.
42. Taylor M. Improving access to dental services for individuals with developmental disabilities. California legislative analyst's office. 2018. Available at: https://lao.ca.gov/reports/2018/3884/dental-for-developmentally-disabled-092718.pdf. Accessed September 27, 2021.
43. Vo AT, Casamassimo PS, Peng J, et al. Denial of operating room access for pediatric dental treatment: a national survey. Pediatr Dent 2021;43(1):33–41.
44. Agency for Healthcare Research and Quality. National healthcare quality and disparities report: chartbook on person- and family-centered care. 2016. AHRQ Pub. No. 16(17)-0015-9-EF. Available at. https://www.ahrq.gov/sites/default/files/wysiwyg/research/findings/nhqrdr/chartbooks/personcentered/qdr2015-chartbook-personcenteredcare.pdf. Accessed September 27, 2021.
45. Hassouneh-Phillips D, McNeff E, Powers L, et al. Invalidation: a central process underlying maltreatment of women with disabilities. Women Health 2005;41(1):33–50.
46. Disability Rights Education and Defense Fund. Healthcare stories. Available at: https://dredf.org/healthcare-stories/. Accessed September 27, 2021.
47. Wilson NJ, Lin Z, Villarosa A, et al. Countering the poor oral health of people with intellectual and developmental disability: a scoping literature review. BMC Public Health 2019;19(1):1530.
48. National Council on Disability. Issue brief. Neglected for too long: dental care for people with intellectual and developmental disabilities. 2017. Available at: https://ncd.gov/sites/default/files/NCD_Dental%20Brief%202017_508.pdf. Accessed September 27, 2021.
49. Queirós FC, Wehby GL, Halpern CT. Developmental disabilities and socioeconomic outcomes in young adulthood. Public Health Rep 2015;130(3):213–21.
50. Zajacova A, Lawrence EM. The relationship between education and health: reducing disparities through a contextual approach. Annu Rev Public Health 2018;39:273–89.
51. Montez JK, Zajacova A, Hayward MD. Disparities in disability by educational attainment across US states. Am J Public Health 2017;107(7):1101–8.
52. Robert Wood Johnson Foundation. Life expectancy: could where you live influence how long you live? 2021. Available at: https://www.rwjf.org/en/library/interactives/whereyouliveaffectshowlongyoulive.html. Accessed September 27, 2021.

53. Rura N. Significant disparities in U.S. life expectancy found at census-tract level. 2020. Available at: https://www.hsph.harvard.edu/news/press-releases/significant-disparities-in-u-s-life-expectancy-found-at-census-tract-level/. Accessed September 27, 2021.
54. A position paper from the Academy of Dentistry for Persons with Disabilities. Preservation of quality oral health care services for people with developmental disabilities. Spec Care Dentist 1998;18(5):180–2.
55. Oktay JS, Tompkins CJ. Personal assistance providers' mistreatment of disabled adults. Health Soc Work 2004;29(3):177–88.
56. Rich AJ, DiGregorio N, Strassle C. Trauma-informed care in the context of intellectual and developmental disability services: perceptions of service providers [published online ahead of print, 2020 Apr 22]. J Intellect Disabil 2020; 1744629520918086.
57. Pulrang A. How to do something good in the disability community if you're not disabled. Forbes. 2020. Available at: https://www.forbes.com/sites/andrewpulrang/2020/12/16/how-to-do-something-good-in-the-disability-community-if-youre-not-disabled/?sh=356eacf47d7f. Accessed September 27, 2021.

From Restraint to Medical Immobilization/Protective Stabilization

Steven P. Perlman, DDS, MScD, DHL (hon), DABSCD[a],*,
Allen Wong, DDS, EdD, DABSCD[b,1],
H. Barry Waldman, DDS, MPH, PhD[c,2], Clive Friedman, BDS[d,3],
Jessica Webb, DDS, MSD, MA, MSRT[e,4], Rick Rader, MD[f,5],
Ray A. Lyons, DDS, DABSCD[g,6]

KEYWORDS

- Restraint • Medical immobilization/protective stabilization • Behavior guidance

KEY POINTS

- There is a hierarchy of behavior guidance techniques that may be necessary to use in treating a patient with a developmental disorder.
- The authors represent the history of how the use of the term restraint for noncompliant or precooperative patients with behavioral issues morphed into the current practice of medical immobilization/protective stabilization.
- The American Academy of Developmental Medicine and Dentistry has created a well-researched and documented policy statement for both physicians and dentists in the case of medical immobilization/protective stabilization for medically necessary health care.

[a] Special Olympics Special Smiles, Boston University Goldman School of Dental Medicine, Penn Dental Medicine; [b] AEGD Program, University of the Pacific Arthur A. Dugoni School of Dentistry, San Francisco, CA 94116, USA; [c] Department of General Dentistry, School of Dental Medicine, Stony Brook University, NY, USA; [d] Cert. Pediatric Dentistry/ Diplomate AAPD, Schulich School of Medicine and Dentistry; [e] Department of Pediatric Dentistry, University of Washington, Advanced Education in Pediatric Dentistry, Postdoctoral Residency Programs, NYU Langone Dental Medicine; [f] Human Development, University of Tennessee/ Chattanooga; [g] Dental Hygiene and Residency Program, University of New Mexico
[1] Present address: 5 Cragmont Avenue, San Francisco, CA 94116.
[2] Present address: 122 Santa Barbara Drive, Plainview, NY 11803.
[3] Present address: 389 Hyde Park Road, London Ontario n6H3r8, Canada.
[4] Present address: Childrens Village, 3801 Kern Road, Yakima, WA 98902.
[5] Present address: 4274 Lake Shore Lane #200, Chattanooga, TN 37415.
[6] Present address: 7316 Carson TRL NW Albuquerque, NM 87120.
* Corresponding author. 500 Puritan Road, Swampscott, MA 01907.
E-mail address: sperlman@bu.edu

Dent Clin N Am 66 (2022) 261–275
https://doi.org/10.1016/j.cden.2022.01.005
0011-8532/22/© 2022 Elsevier Inc. All rights reserved.

dental.theclinics.com

Making the case for medical immobilization/protective stabilization (MI/PS) can sometimes be best exemplified through practical examples. Here are just a few after best efforts of behavioral guidance are exhausted.

Practical examples
1. A 4-year-old child with special needs falls and vertically fractures both primary maxillary central incisors. The child is extremely uncooperative, and the teeth are nonrestorable. The child is in constant pain, needs to be medically immobilized for the examination, and it is impossible to obtain radiographs. The treatment is extraction of the fractured incisors. How will you treat the patient immediately to relieve the pain and what behavioral guidance techniques will you need to use?
2. A 16-year-old teenager with a disability, uncooperative, combative, presents with a history of pain for a week. The only safe way to do a full examination is to use MI/PS. He is not eating or sleeping. Clinical examination revealed a deep carious lesion on tooth number 29.
   It appears to be restorable, maybe even requiring a stainless-steel crown. Other carious lesions are present. How will you provide relief of pain at the visit and help the patient who has suffered for a week?
3. A 45-year-old person with special needs residing in a group home presents with advanced periodontal disease, pain, and infection.

Clinical examination using MI/PS demonstrates the problem is clearly from nonrestorable periodontally involved molars.

The patient has not been eating, sleeping, and exhibiting aggressive and combative behavior to his staff and fellow residents of the home.

What do you tell them and their direct support professionals?

In all these case scenarios, the patients have moderate to profound intellectual disabilities, multiple comorbidities, and no contraindications to MI/PS, sedation, or general anesthesia (GA).

At the chairside visit, how do you and will you provide treatment to relieve pain and control infection? How long do you keep them on medications? How long do they need to wait for care?

What will you recommend to the patient/parent or guardian? We hope after reading this article that you learned that MI/PS is the safest, most immediate, and maybe the only behavioral guidance technique available to you to relieve the pain, suffering, and overall health of your patient instead of delaying medically necessary dental care.

There is not a more controversial issue than MI/PS in the pediatric or adult world, for both neurotypical and patients with special health care needs. Restraint is a term formerly used that currently has negative connotations in the United States and global community.[1–8]

For the purpose of this article, we will limit its scope to children and adults with physical and intellectual disabilities in the United States and Canada.

Patients with special needs often present with unique challenges to the dental team.[2]

They may have a wide range of medical conditions ranging from minor health issues to the most severe and complex medical problems someone could possibly have.

They often have behavioral considerations ranging from completely cooperative to as uncooperative, dangerous, or combative as a patient can be, sometimes creating a potentially harmful situation.

The pediatric literature is robust in providing information on basic behavioral support techniques, but there exists a paucity of information about adult patients.

As eloquently stated by one of our authors, "Although this segment of our population often poses a unique debate to all members of the healthcare team, few disciplines face the extremely delicate and exigent task required in dentistry."[2]

"Clinical dental treatment is the most exacting and demanding medical procedure that persons with special needs undergo on a regular basis throughout their lifetime. Dental treatment is basically surgical in nature, usually requiring controlled placement of sharpened instrumentation in intimate proximity to the face, airway, and highly vascularized and innervated oral tissues."[2]

This article will also try to address why the issue of MI/PS is really not a problem for our medical colleagues but has become a significant barrier in access to care for oral health providers.

We will review the ethical and practical use of the current MI/PS policy and see how medicine addresses the use of medical immobilization.

If a child who cannot sit still, falls and has an injury, there is no hesitation to medically immobilize a child for radiographs or treatment.

So why is there such an aversion when it comes to oral care?

CURRENT MI/PS POLICY

According to the American Academy of Developmental Medicine and Dentistry Guidelines (AADMD) 2017[9], protective stabilization or immobilization is defined as "any manual method, physical or mechanical device, material, or equipment that immobilizes or reduces the ability of a patient to move his or her arms, legs, body, or head freely."[9–13]

Consistent with the United Nation's principles for the *"Protection of Persons with Mental Illness and Care and principles Least Intrusiveness and Least Restrictiveness*, and as may be indicated with any patient, techniques that serve to desensitize a patient should always be employed prior to consideration of the use of stabilization, immobilization or bracing of people." Furthermore, a full range of person-centered positive behavioral supports must be considered and used with people before, during, and after any application of stabilization, immobilization, or bracing.

Historically and now, there is substantial debate over the philosophy and clinical wisdom of using GA or intravenous (IV) sedation for general dentistry for patients with intellectual and developmental disabilities (IDD). Notwithstanding, GA or IV sedation must be considered as part of the continuum of medical immobilization, and then only when clinically indicated.

PRINCIPLES AND CORE VALUES

- The full array of positive behavioral supports should be considered before, during, and after the application of stabilization techniques.
- Protective stabilization should, to the extent possible, be person-centered and conducted in a fashion that maintains the patients' privacy and dignity.
- Protective stabilization should be provided in the least restrictive manner possible.
- Staff should be trained in the safe, efficacious employment of any devices, techniques, or protocols. Their training requires documentation and evidence of competency-based training with refresher training based on the frequency of use of stabilization techniques, confidence level, and self-assessment, but no less frequently than every 2 years.
- Patients should be monitored (health status) during and after the use of any protective stabilization.

- The use of protective stabilization requires documentation and should include the reason for the stabilization, any alternatives that were tried (where possible), members of the health care provider team, outcomes, and any recommendations for future use of the stabilization protocols with this patient.
- Obtain informed consent/assent. Communicate the intention to use protective stabilization to the patients, parents, family members, legal guardians/conservators, direct care staff, and others responsible for their custody and care at the first available opportunity. Provide them with the rationale, risks, consequences, and expectations. Document the dialogue. (If the person is receiving long term services and supports, it is likely appropriate to review any recommended use of stabilization with the person's interdisciplinary team. In addition, laws and applicable regulations should be consulted for involvement of human rights committees or their equivalent.)[14–18]

RATIONALE

The AADMD believes that all individuals with IDD deserve the highest quality of medical and dental care.

To achieve that goal, it is imperative that the clinician understands the cognitive, behavioral, sensory, reasoning, and experiential histories of the patient. There will be circumstances where it is reasonable to expect that a patient may not present as a cooperative, compliant, and optimal patient. (See WHO Manual on Mental Health Law and Human Rights and Quality Rights.) Should there be a risk of the patient becoming agitated, unsteady, thrashing, contorted, flailing, and spasmodic, which has the potential for an unsuccessful outcome of the procedure with unhealthy consequences, and/or the procedure has to be repeated or the results compromised, the AADMD believes measured interventions that increase the opportunity for a successful procedure with a successful outcome is preferred to going to the surgical suite for GA with all the inherent risks that provides. Sir William Osler, the doyen of American medicine observed, *"Do the kindest thing and do it first"* Often the kindest (and safest) thing is to stabilize and immobilize the patient to ensure a clinically successful procedure.

INDICATIONS

Protective stabilization is indicated when:

- A patient requires diagnosis and/or treatment and cannot be safely examined and/or treated without stabilization.
- Medical or dental treatment is needed, and uncontrolled movements risk the safety of the patient, staff, dentist, physician, nurse, aide, or parent without the use of protective stabilization.
- A previously cooperative patient quickly becomes agitated during the appointment, to protect their safety and help to expedite completion of treatment.
- A sedated patient may become unexpectedly active during treatment.
- A patient with special health care needs may experience uncontrolled movements that would be harmful or significantly interfere with the quality of care.[19]

BENEFITS

When used correctly and in accordance with these guidelines, protective stabilization provides the following benefits:

- Provides the clinician with (as near as possible) an examination and operating field with a reduction in untoward movements.
- Provides protection for the patient and the health care team.
- Provides the patient with a familiarity of expectations which can diminish future anxiety promoting health care visits.

CONTRAINDICATIONS

Protective stabilization is contraindicated for:

- Compliant and cooperative nonsedated patients.
- Patients with medical, dental, psychological, sensory, behavioral, psychiatric, or physical conditions that prevent them from being safely immobilized.
- Patients with a history of significant physical or psychological trauma due to previous restraints (unless no other alternatives are available).

EQUIPMENT

Numerous devices are available to achieve protective stabilization (medical immobilization). The staff should be knowledgeable regarding the ideal characteristics of the devices they will be using; these devices should be:

- Easily used
- Appropriately sized for the patient
- Soft and contoured to minimize potential injury to and provide comfort to the patient
- Specifically designed for patient stabilization (no improvised equipment)
- Able to be sanitized and disinfected after each use.
- Mouth props may be used for oral and dental procedures as an immobilization device. The use of a mouth prop in a compliant patient is not considered protective stabilization.
- Hand guarding (the use of the clinician's hands and arms or that of the assistant) to provide adjunct stabilization can be used providing that at no time the hand guarding should restrict blood flow or respiration.

HISTORICAL PERSPECTIVE

At the request of countless health care providers, in 2016, Dr Rick Rader was tasked by the American Academy of Developmental Medicine and Dentistry (AADMD) to come up with guidelines and a policy statement on MI/PS for people with intellectual and physical disabilities that would be interdisciplinary, evidence-based, and inclusive of all age groups including children and adults.

The Creation and Adoption of the AADMD's Policy Statement on Immobilization and Stabilization: The Case for Equity with Dentistry.

Rick Rader, MD, FAAIDD, FAADM, DHL (hon)

Dr Rader writes:

As a medical student, I performed my pediatric rotation at London's famed Hospital for Sick Children (The Great Ormond Street Hospital).

One afternoon in the emergency room, I was handed a card as I was summoned into cubicle 4. The "casualty card" simply read, "FOLNC" it was shorthand for Foreign Object in Left Nasal Cavity. Although that was an appropriate note, I enjoyed the history (or as they currently say, "the narrative"). Mathew was a 4-year-old boy who somehow managed to stick the left front wheel of his 1981 red Scammell lodged up his nose.

This was not hard to do for a wheel the size of a button. The wheel was from Mathew's favorite Matchbox scale model toy truck.

Dr Nedwaite, one of the teachers, instructed me to have Mathew sit on my lap and wrap my arms around his torso while he extracted the truck's wheel. Mathew was happy to be able to remount the wheel on his Matchbox toy. That was my earliest introduction to immobilization. As we were leaving the cubicle, Dr Nedwaite said, "In the States they would call that immobilization," here we just call it "holding the lad so we can pluck out the wheel." I was sold.

I had also seen immobilization (also known as procedural stabilization) used in a variety of settings for a variety of reasons; all geared to insuring the best clinical outcomes for patients who because of communication, behavioral, sensory, neuromotor control, anxiety, and other conditions required limbs, torso, and head movements to be controlled. Clinicians need a secure anatomic field to enable them to safely and effectively suture, draw blood, palpate, insert an IV line, remove a foreign object, and perform dozens of other necessary procedures that sudden movements would prove dangerous. The alternative of sending individuals to the operating room under GA is contraindicated because of the risk, expense, availability, and medical necessity. In the case of dental procedures, the need for a stable and steady operative field is even compounded. Drills moving at 400,000 rpm, injections and probes can suddenly be weaponized without warning when a patient jerks his or her head back and forth. The use of both immobilization techniques and sedation can often be minimized or avoided when a program of desensitization is used and is made part of an individual's behavior plan. Desensitization is not feasible when an acute procedure is required.

Wherever possible the employment of an approved desensitization program is always preferred to other stabilizing maneuvers. His career path brought him into the field of developmental medicine (the medical treatment of individuals with IDD).

I was made aware of several cases where dentists using assistants to immobilize patients with IDD were accused and charged with assault, restraint, and imprisonment. They were investigated by the state dental board where their licenses were suspended during the course of the investigation. Many of these cases dragged on for months and both the loss of income and the legal expenses easily convinced these dentists not to welcome patients with ID/DD back into their practices. No one can appreciate the stress these dentists experienced by accusations of abuse. These cases also served as the rationale for dentists to refuse to treat these vulnerable patients.

The identical immobilization practices used by physicians in emergency rooms, clinics, offices, and hospitals were acknowledged as appropriate, beneficial, and required. One would be hard-pressed to find lawsuits or medical board investigations directed at emergency room physicians who had an assistant hold a patient's arm while they started an IV line.

Dr Rader believed that in both medical and dental settings, the use of immobilization policies and procedures should be equally understood, respected, supported, and encouraged.

There are numerous medical specialty associations that have policies that dictate the use of these stabilizing procedures including several radiology academies, orthopedic groups, the American College of Emergency Physicians, and the American Academy of Pediatrics among others. I contacted the American College of Emergency Physicians and requested that "dental procedures" be added to their indications for the appropriate use of medical immobilization. After months of review, they decided not to add that term to their policy.

It was at this time that Dr Rader (VP for Public Policy and Advocacy) understood that the American Academy of Developmental Medicine and Dentistry (www.aadmd.org) had to take the leading role in creating a set of policies and procedures that would recognize that a single set of guidelines should be applicable to both the medical and dental domains.

A rigorous review of numerous immobilization policies was evaluated, assessed, and placed in various scenarios that would be applied to patients with IDD. Over the course of 6 months, the draft of the proposed policy was reviewed by clinicians, nurses, advocates, self-advocates, behaviorists, human rights committees, families, medical ethicists, administrators, attorneys, and hospital patient safety groups.

We believe the AADMD's Immobilization and Stabilization Policies and Procedures represents the collective wisdom, sensitivity, and experience of the above-respected stakeholders. The policy was created and approved as a living and evolving document and the AADMD is posed to address and consider new evidence that would impact on the improvement of the policy.

CONCERNS OF MI/PS

What has changed in the past 3 decades that has made access to care for children and adults with disabilities more difficult than ever before.

There are many contributing factors that have negatively changed the landscape.

Historically, pediatric dentists have always been the providers for both children and adults with physical and intellectual disabilities. In 1940, the American Board of Pedodontics was established but the Academy of Pedodontics was not created until 1947.[20]

In 1994, the specialty became age-defined and over the years there has been a movement to lower the age limit of patients they treat, and transitioning to adult practices is now occurring at the age of 14 or even as young as the eruption of the first permanent molars.

The academy's marketing initiative, originating years ago refers to themselves as "the big authority on little teeth." Even their daily online communication is called "little teeth chat."

Children's hospitals throughout the country were known to provide a safe haven for adults with special needs but no longer are encouraged to accept patients over the age of 18 or 21 years.

After graduation, most pediatric dentists seek employment in wealthy suburbs, rather than inner city or rural areas where the burden of dental disease is much higher. If a program does not teach or encourage MI/PS, the only option is sedation or GA.[3]

There is an enormous lack of qualified faculty in dental and hygiene schools with the knowledge, expertise, and experience to educate students in the care of patients with special needs.[3]

The shift away from MI/PS toward pharmacologic management and techniques such as interim therapeutic restorations are not long-term solutions but symptomatic of a large and concerning problem: the increasing numbers of dental professionals who do not have the education or skills needed to guide the behaviors of children and adults with special health care needs in a positive direction.[3]

There is no substantial didactic or clinical dental curriculum regarding people with disabilities. Financial constraints are often cited as one of the most significant barriers in access to care.[3]

Most of this population relies on Medicaid or other programs whose low levels of reimbursement are one of the reasons for the low numbers of clinicians participating making access to care nearly impossible.

The history of our involvement with "restraint" issues in dentistry dates back to the mid-1970s, involving The Academy of Dentistry for the Handicapped and The American Academy of Pediatric Dentistry.

"Restraint" came under the topic of Behavior Management and was addressed in symposiums and the literature. There were hardly any issues that came to the attention of either organization.[6,7]

The Academy of Dentistry for the Handicapped (ADH), which was founded in 1957, became the Academy of Dentistry for Persons with Disabilities in 1994. Several of us were Board Members at that time and instrumental in the name change.

In 1987, 3 organizations decided they shared similar interests and missions, and merged to become The Federation of Special Care Organizations in Dentistry.

The 3 components were The American Association of Hospital Dentists, The American Association of Geriatric Dentistry, and the Academy of Dentistry for the Handicapped.

A review of the literature on the issue of restraint in Dentistry was almost exclusively in 3 journals: Special Care Dentistry, Pediatric Dentistry, and Dentistry for Children.

In addition, there were symposiums such as Dental Management of the Handicapped Child (1974) at the University of Iowa, Behavior Management for the Pediatric Dental Patient (AAPD IOWA 1998), and Beyond the Guidelines: Factors Affecting Behavior Guidance (AAPD 2013 Chicago) all discussing restraint, sedation, and GA.

To clarify the use of restraints in dentistry and provide guidelines, in 1997, Special Care Dentistry Journal published the ADH ad hoc committee report: The use of restraints in the delivery of dental care for the handicapped legal, ethical and medical considerations.

ABSTRACT

Presented is the final report of the Ad Hoc Committee on the Use of Physical Restraints. The report discusses legal, ethical, and medical issues of physical restraint of patients. Conclusions included: there is no consensus among the states on definition of restraint–dental practitioners should check with their own states for current rulings; the current national view is that restraint should only be used when absolutely necessary, and the least restrictive form should be used, and it shall not be used as punishment or for the convenience of the staff; use of restraint is acceptable dental practice when appropriately used for behavior control of patients with developmentally disabling conditions; documentation is required; physical restraint should cause no physical injury; and informed consent should be used, after checking with authorities as to proper form.[21]

This pioneering article resulted in providing a framework that led to few problems for clinicians utilizing restraint as a behavioral guidance technique to treat patients with behavioral issues, or involuntary movements.

The request for MI/PS often came from the patient, family, or caregivers, as the safest alternative to sedation and GA.

The American Academy of Pediatric Dentistry publishes a biannual Reference Manual defining the scope of Pediatric Dentistry and Clinical practice guidelines that are "statements that include recommendations intended to optimize patient care. They are informed by a systematic review of evidence and an assessment of the benefits and harm of alternative care options."[4,22]

Recommendations on Protective Stabilization were developed by the Council on Clinical Affairs starting in 1996 and adopted in 2013 and revised in 2017.

These guidelines created a new landscape and were very controversial, greatly affected clinical practice in a negative way and were not evidence-based but created to stop the negative perception that corporate dentistry was strapping children down to do multiple quadrants of restorative dentistry in one setting.

These new guidelines on Protective Stabilization defined it as an advanced behavior guidance technique along with sedation and GA. In addition, it went on to say its use was beyond the core knowledge students receive in predoctoral dental education.

"Dentists considering the use of these advanced behavior guidance should seek additional training through a residency program, a graduate program, and/or an extensive continuing education course that involves both didactic and experiential mentored training."

Throughout the history presented, the glaring problem has been that the only guidelines on MI/PS were created by the AAPD and did not address patients in late adolescence and adults, especially for those with IDD.

In 2002, the American Academy of Developmental Medicine and Dentistry was founded by a group of physicians and dentists, including several authors of this article.

A true interdisciplinary organization composed of leading educators and clinicians specializing in patients with IDD and physical disabilities, the AADMD has become the leading organization in policy, advocacy, education, and standards of care.

Behavioral issues are the cornerstone of pediatric dentistry or for those treating adolescents and adults with disabilities. It is a significant barrier to care, even more important than the level of training and education of the provider, or poor and inadequate reimbursement for services.

The clinician must approach each patient and each visit as a new encounter, without implicit bias, nor a thought of using a referring colleague's experience, or a scale such as The Frankl Behavior Management Scale.[18]

There are literally dozens of reasons for people with disabilities that may cause or affect them to change their acceptance and ability to tolerate dental procedures from one visit to the next or even during the same visit.

They may just be in a bad mood that day, or not received their medications at the appropriate time.

They might not be feeling well at the appointment time and unable to express themselves (ie, constipation or menstrual cramps)

The usual staff person or family member who accompanies them to their health visits may not be with them that day.

They may prefer a male or female provider.

They did not get satisfactory sleep the night before.

They might not like the sound or smell of the office that day.

They may have anxiety beyond what is typical for them.

For children and adults on the Autism Spectrum Disorder, the saying goes "if you've seen one patient with autism, you' ve seen one patient with autism."

Dr Hackie Reitman, Founder and President of Different Brains states, "Every brain is like a snowflake, no two are alike".

Statements like these are so true in the case of developmental health care. Every patient and situation is so different, it is impossible to predict outcomes.

Numerous studies well document the fact that dental and hygiene students receive little if any hands-on training in the care of patients with developmental disorders.[23]

Personal communication between two of the authors (Perlman and Waldman) with CODA members revealed an unwillingness of the schools to address this problem because of a lack of trained faculty members and inadequate compensation in the clinics.

It was only after repeated pressure and years of discussion that CODA passed a resolution in 2007 implementing student competency in diagnosis and treatment planning only for patients with special health care needs.

It also was possible for a dental/hygiene school graduate to complete their education without a single encounter with a patient with a disability.

In the past, behavior management has been the long-standing traditional term used by all health care professionals, direct support personnel, or families to describe how a health provider can deliver services in a safe, appropriate, and competent manner.[6,19,24–29]

In 2006, the American Academy of Pediatric Dentistry officially changed this terminology to reflect nomenclature in the field. Indeed, no one likes to be "managed" but rather supported or guided.

The term "behavior guidance" is thus used to better describe a collaborative philosophy that is person-centered, in that it considers the individual, evaluates his or her environment, support, resources, and attempts to plan how challenging behavior can be moderated.

Regarding behavior guidance as an essential technique, there is a hierarchy of treatment strategies for dental professionals to use to assist patients in their attempt to cope with clinical oral health treatment.

The literature is abundant with quality articles and books but mostly in the pediatric world.

The most important considerations as previously stated are that every patient and visit is unique and a very personal exchange between themselves and the dental professional.

That it is up to the clinician how to approach each situation.

It is important for the clinician to be in their "comfort zone" based on their training and level of experience.

Past experiences can lead to sound clinical judgment and the more exposure to this population the clinician has, the better they will become.

The philosophy the clinician must adhere to is that care should be rendered in the least restrictive manner. The techniques may range from Tell-Show-Do, to MI/PS, to sedation and GA.

Polypharmacy, genetics, past and current medical history, and adverse childhood experiences by the patient can all play a role in decision making.

Other, important issues to consider are:

At what level do we decide what is medically necessary dental/health care?

Is delaying treatment or supervised neglect ethical or acceptable?

Regarding the AAPD guidelines how does MI/PS cause loss of dignity without any evidence-based literature, or falsely described "toxic stress."

How can one justify doing sedation or GA without a thorough oral examination?

How can the clinician justify sedation or GA for an oral prophylaxis, simple restorative or surgical procedure that can be accomplished safely and efficiently with MI/PS?

How can an educator endorsed by the AAPD declare "But the last time I looked at my degree was D.D.S. (Dr of Dental Surgery), not Dr of Psychology.[30]

That MI/PS is most often used to secure the noncompliant patient and as cooperation is often achieved it can be used with less or no restrictions on the arms, legs, or torso.

CONCERNS FOR HOSPITAL AND OFFICE CONSCIOUS SEDATION

The use of the hospital operating room for dental cases has been severely curtailed by the pandemic.

The growing numbers and lack of reimbursement to hospitals will continue to be difficult for providers to secure hospital time.

The dramatic and unconscionable overuse of GA is now hurting the profession.[1]

How can the clinician look at a patient, family member, or caregiver in the eyes and say yes, your loved one needs treatment but there is a 1- to 3-year wait for a GA case.

Can anyone argue that MI/PS is not the safest alternative to sedation and GA.

That although the profession claims safety and lack of accidental deaths and untoward reactions, there is no available data to support or substantiate it.

In fact, accidents, brain damage, and deaths in many instances occur in dental offices.

However, the truth is for any patient, the actual pronouncement of death occurs mostly in hospital emergency rooms in the presence of a physician. A critical situation can possibly occur in the dental operatory, ambulatory care, or surgicenter.

The call is made to 911, and however the condition of the patient the decision is made in the hospital, therefore there are no data on in-office complications.

More and more research has shown the negative effects of GA agents, especially repeated exposure on developing cerebral tissue.

Essential Techniques of Behavioral Support

Voice control
Nonverbal communication
Tell show do
Positive reinforcement
Contingent escape
Noncontingent escape
Distraction
Parental presence/absence
Modeling
Shaping
Flexibility
Consistency
Desensitization
Repetitive tasking
Hypnosis
Escape extinction
Flooding or systemic desensitization
Alternative behavior strategies
Sensory adapted environment
Aroma therapy
Social stories
Teacch—Treatment and Education of Autism and related Communication-handicapped Children
PECs—Picture Exchange Communication System
Sensory integration
Music therapy
Craniosacral therapy
Equine therapy

Advanced Behavioral Techniques

Hand over mouth exercise or (aversive conditioning)
MI/PS
Sedation
General anesthesia[2,31]

The Centers for Medicare and Medicaid Services defines physical restraint as"(A) Any manual method, physical or mechanical device, material, or equipment that immobilizes or reduces the ability of a patient to move his or her arms, legs, body, or head freely; or (B) A drug or medication when it is used as a restriction to manage the patient' s behavior or restrict the patient's freedom of movement and is not a standard treatment or dosage for the patient's condition."[32,33]

This definition clearly has limitations when applied directly to dentistry "as it does not accurately or comprehensively reflect the indications or utilization of restraint in dentistry".[4]

Active immobilization involves restraint by another person such as the parent, dentist, or auxiliary.[4,10]

Passive immobilization uses a restraining device. Socioeconomic status, geographic location, and ethnic/cultural differences of patients and their parents may influence parental preferences for behavioral guidance techniques.[4,10]

Thus far, education has offered limited exposure. In 2007, a predoctoral dental school survey demonstrated 27% of programs provided "No clinical experience on the use of an immobilization device".[4,17]

Is not swaddling a newborn a form of medical immobilization? Every baby leaves a hospital swaddled.

The calming and comforting benefit of swaddling, which is the age-old practice of wrapping infants in blankets, have been traditionally used in multiple cultures. Modern applications may enhance an infant's sleep, limit crying, and also can include prescribed use to reduce pain during medical procedures such as blood draws. The benefits of swaddling may persist throughout a lifetime, as therapists are finding that deep pressure stimulation to be useful in managing anxiety, post-traumatic stress, insomnia, chronic fatigue, and other mental health issues. Deep pressure slows heart rate, improves circulation, and allows muscles to relax. It seems to increase the body's own release of endorphins, serotonin, dopamine, and possibly melatonin.

These "feel good" neurotransmitters support impulse control, attention, social behavior, and sleep.

Cradle boards have been used by indigenous peoples in North America and Scandinavia to this day. "Papoose" is a traditional word referring to a baby or young Native American child and is intended to be used as a term of endearment.

Patients undergoing sedation and GA tend to receive more extensive restorative treatment than necessary.

The justification from the clinician is that patients who require advanced behavioral techniques are at a higher risk for dental disease and therefore need more extensive, and more costly treatment to obviate future needs.

ABOUT THE AUTHORS

The 6 authors have a collective career of almost 300 years immersed in the medical and dental care of children and adults with intellectual and developmental disorders. They have practiced in institutions, private sectors, public health clinics, and all have academic appointments. They are all or were trench warriors whose philosophies and techniques are the result of tens of thousands of patient visits who have intellectual and physical disabilities and the thousands of health professional students and residents who they trained. They have held leadership positions in many professional organizations, created and implemented local and global programs, and have made significant contributions to the health care of children and adults with disabilities.

Together they have published over 2000 articles, significantly contributing to the body of literature on special patient care, lectured at countless major dental and medical meetings, testified before congressional hearings, and met with politicians from all over the world.

They decided to band together to provide dental and hygiene professionals with an evidence-based, practical, realistic, comprehensive, well-referenced review, and recommendation for the use of MI/PS as the safest alternative to sedation and GA for many situations.

CLINICS CARE POINTS

- AADMD guidelines for medical immobilization/protective stabilization are evidence-based and the only guidelines recommended equally for physicians, dentists, and other interdisciplinary professions.
- MI/PS must be considered as the safest alternative to sedation and general anesthesia for the precooperative and uncooperative patients with developmental disabilities.
- Predoctoral dental education does not have a comprehensive curriculum in Special Patient Care.
- People with intellectual disabilities are the most medically and dentally underserved population.
- Oral health is the most unmet health care need for children, adolescents, and adults with intellectual and physical disabilities.
- There are many barriers to dental care for people with developmental disabilities; behaviors being a major reason for dental professionals' unwillingness to treat this population.

DISCLOSURE

The authors have nothing to disclose.

REFERENCES

1. Chavis SE, Wu E, Munz SM. Considerations for protective stabilization in community general dental practice for adult patients with special healthcare needs. Compend Contin Educ Dent 2021;42(3):134–8.
2. Raposa KA, Perlman SP. Treating the Dental Patient with a Developmental Disorder. Wiley-Blackwell; 2012.
3. Killian MK, Kupietzky A, Croll T. Teaching behavior management of pediatric dental patients. are we off track. Inside Dentistry 2020;16(2).
4. American Academy of Pediatric Dentistry TRMoPD. Use of Protective Stabilization for pediatric dental patients; 2020.
5. Nelson TM, Sheller B, Friedman CS, et al. Educational and therapeutic behavioral approaches to providing dental care for patients with Autism Spectrum Disorder. Spec Care Dentist 2015;35(3):105–13.
6. Nathan JE. Behavioral management strategies for young pediatric dental patients with disabilities. ASDC J Dent Child 2001;68(2):89–101.
7. Oueis HS, Ralstrom E, Miriyala V, et al. Alternatives for hand over mouth exercise after its elimination from the clinical guidelines of the american academy of pediatric dentistry. Pediatr Dent 2010;32(3):223–8.

8. Bridgman AM, Wilson MA. The treatment of adult patients with a mental disability. Br Dental J 2000;189:195–8.
9. Townsend JA. Dental Care for Children with Special Needs: Protective Stabilization in the Dental Setting. Switzerland: Springer Nature Switzerland AG; 2019.
10. Manual AR. Behavior Guidance for the Pediatric Dental Patient; 2020.
11. Karibe H, Umezu Y, Hasegawa Y, et al. Factors affecting the use of protective stabilization in dental patients with cognitive disabilities. Spec Care Dentist 2008; 28(5):214–20.
12. Marty M, Marquet A, Valera MC. Perception of protective stabilization by pediatric dentists: a qualitative study. JDR Clin Trans Res 2020. 2380084420963933.
13. Davis DM, Fadavi S, Kaste LM, et al. Acceptance and use of protective stabilization devices by pediatric dentistry diplomates in the United States. J Dent Child (Chic) 2016;83(2):60–6.
14. Ilha MC, Feldens CA, Razera J, et al. Protective stabilization in pediatric dentistry: a qualitative study on the perceptions of mothers, psychologists, and pediatric dentists. Int J Paediatr Dent 2020;1–10.
15. Kemp F. Alternatives: a review of non-pharmacologic approaches to increasing the cooperation of patients with special needs to inherently unpleasant dental procedures. Behav Analyst Today 2005;6(2):88–108.
16. Strange DM. The evolution of behavior guidance: a history of professional, practice, corporate and societal influences. Pediatr Dent 2014;36(2):128–31.
17. Kupietzky A. Treating very young patients with conscious sedation and medical immobilization: a Jewish perspective. Alpha Omegan 2005;98(4):33–7.
18. Frankl SN, Shiere FR, Fogels HR. Should the parent remain with the child in the dental operatory? J Dentistry Child 1962;29:150–63.
19. AADMD. Medical Immobilization Procedure Stabilization. August 2017 ed. AADMD website: AADMD; 2017.
20. Dentistry AAoP. Five Decades of Excellence; 1997.
21. Fenton SJ, Fenton LI+, Kimmelman BB, et al. ADH ad hoc committee report: The use of restraints in the delivery of dental care for the handicapped—legal, ethical, and medical considerations. Spec Care Dentist 1987;7(6):253–6.
22. American Academy of Pediatric Dentistry TRMoPD. Behavior Guidance for the Pediatric Dental Patient. Chicago, IL; 2020;292–310.
23. Casamassimo P, Berlocher WC, Cheney W, et al. The future of pediatric dentistry advanced education: the need for change in training standards. Pediatr Dent 2009;31(4):298–309.
24. de Castro AM, de Oliveira FS, de Paiva Novaes MS, et al. Behavior guidance techniques in pediatric dentistry: attitudes of parents of children with disabilities and without disabilities. Spec Care Dentist 2013;33(5):213–7.
25. Martinez Mier EA, Walsh CR, Farah CC, et al. Acceptance of behavior guidance techniques used in pediatric dentistry by parents from diverse backgrounds. Clin Pediatr (Phila) 2019;58(9):977–84.
26. Wright GZ, Kupietzky A. Behavior Management in Dentistry for Children. 2nd edition. John Wiley& Sons, Inc; 2014.
27. Lyons RA. Understanding basic behavioral support techniques as an alternative to sedation and anesthesia. Spec Care Dentist 2009;29(1):39–50.
28. Connick C, Palat M, Pugliese S. The appropriate use of physical restraint: considerations. ASDC J Dent Child 2000;4:256–62, 31.
29. Curzon ME. Strap him down or knock him out: Is conscious sedation with restraint an alternative to general anaesthesia? Br Dent J 2004;196(12):732 [discussion: 32–3].

30. Chat AOCLT. Americas Pediatric Dentists. The Big Authority on Little Teeth; 2020.
31. Romer M. Consent, restraint, and people with special needs: a review. Spec Care Dentist 2009;29(1):58–66.
32. Services CfMaM. H.H.S. 2012;S.482.13:9-13.
33. Medical Immobilization: Authority IC FMR Regulation 242, 244,245. Medical Immobilization: Restraint Use in State Operated Developmental Centers and Programs; 2005.

The Prenatal Diagnosis and Consultation for Cleft Lip and Palate Prior to Presurgical Infant Orthopedics and Early Dental Care

Brett Chiquet, DDS, PhD[a], Lizbeth Holguin, DDS[b],*

KEYWORDS

- Cleft lip and palate • Nasoalveolar molding • Dental home
- Presurgical infant orthopedic

KEY POINTS

- Prenatal consultation is important to minimize the stress associated with the diagnosis.
- Infants born with cleft lip and/or cleft palate should have surgical, dental, and therapy that start in infancy and continue to adulthood.
- Infants born with cleft lip and/or cleft palate may benefit from nasoalveolar molding therapy before surgery to minimize the severity of the birth defect.
- Children born with cleft lip and/or cleft palate have unique dental needs and should establish a dental home by their first birthday to coordinate dental care/treatments throughout childhood and adolescence.

The news of expecting a child in most cases comes with great joy and stress from both parents but specially from the expecting mother. Great anticipation can surround the prenatal anatomy ultrasound scans as the expectant parents are excited to "see" their child for the first time. Once the intrauterine diagnosis of cleft lip with or without cleft palate (CL/P) is confirmed by ultrasound (**Fig. 1**) is often a shock for families facing this and must be addressed with empathy in a comprehensive and coordinated way to provide the family with the correct information to make informed decisions on the child's behalf. Therefore, appropriate management of the expectant mother with a positive diagnosis of CL/P best provides the necessary information and anticipation to lower the stress factor during pregnancy.

[a] Department of Pediatric Dentistry, UTHealth, The University of Texas Health Science Center at Houston, School of Dentistry; [b] Division Chief of Pediatric/Hospital Dentistry, El Paso Children's Hospital
* Corresponding author.
E-mail address: lizbeth.holguin@gmail.com

Dent Clin N Am 66 (2022) 277–281
https://doi.org/10.1016/j.cden.2022.01.007
0011-8532/22/© 2022 Elsevier Inc. All rights reserved.

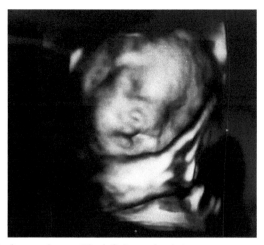

Fig. 1. Ultrasound of an embryo with cleft lip and palate.

During the prenatal screening of pregnant women, fetal anomalies requiring surgery may be diagnosed. Health care providers should have a basic knowledge of these diseases, including their workup, comorbidities, prognosis, treatment options, and any considerations that need to be made in planning for birth.[1] Preparations should be made to ensure sufficient resources are available at the location of birth.

Successful management of the child born with a CL/P requires coordinated care provided by a number of different specialties including oral/maxillofacial surgery, otolaryngology, genetics/dysmorphology, speech/language pathology, orthodontics, pediatric dentistry, prosthodontics, pediatric surgery, pediatric otolaryngology, and others.[2] For this reason, appropriate management of the prenatal consultation with a multidisciplinary team is of extreme importance.

When indicated, referrals should be made to different specialists, especially when the option of presurgical infant orthopedic appliance therapy (PSIO) is recommended.

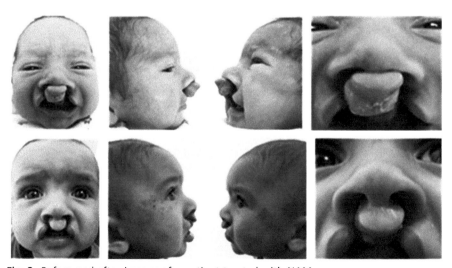

Fig. 2. Before and after images of a patient treated with NAM.

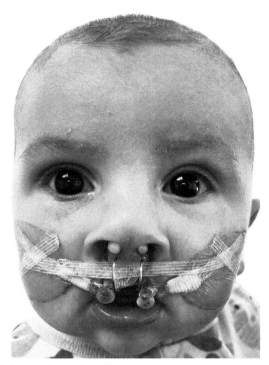

Fig. 3. Picture of infant with NAM appliance.

Consultation with an appropriate dental specialist should be made for cleft lip taping and or presurgical orthopedics including, but not limited to, nasoalveolar molding (NAM). A craniofacial orthodontist, pediatric dentist (or appropriately-trained clinician) who can discuss with the family the types of infant orthopedic services available and the rationale for using infant orthopedics before initial cleft lip repair is necessary.[3]

Prenatal consultation should be individualized to meet the specific needs of each patient and family.

The prenatal consultation involving the treatment of NAM includes:

- In-person consultation to present the expecting parents with comprehensive, in-depth information about NAM therapy for the child with cleft lip and palate
- Encourage parents to communicate with pediatrician/primary care provider and have a birth plan
- Selection of birth hospital predelivery
- Explain cleft care timeline
- Discuss options for breastfeeding and express breast milk
- Offer to network with other families that have gone thru PSIO
- Provide insurance information and codes

PRESURGICAL INFANT ORTHOPEDICS, NASOALVEOLAR MOLDING

Presurgical infant orthopedics has been described since the 1950s in multiple articles and its benefits have been well documented in the literature. When considering nasoalveolar molding (NAM), the optimal time for the first evaluation is within the first few weeks of life and, whenever possible, within the first few days,[3] due to the time sensitivity nature of this therapy. NAM takes the advantage of the flexibility of the cartilaginous septum in the first few weeks after birth. The high levels of hyaluronic acid ,increases the malleability of immature cartilage and its ability to maintain a permanent correction of its form. In addition, the ability to nonsurgically construct the columella through the application of tissue expansion principles, improves facial esthetics. This construction is performed by gradual elongation of the nasal stents and the application of tissue-expanding elastic forces that are applied to the prolabium. The use of the NAM technique has eliminated surgical columella reconstruction and the resultant scar tissue.[4] As a result of presurgical nasoalveolar molding, the primary surgical repair of the nose and lip heals under minimal tension, thereby reducing scar formation and improving the esthetic result.[5]

Improved primary surgeries result in better outcomes and minimal incidence of revisions, this being the biggest benefit for patients and families of children with cleft lip and palate (Figs. 2 and 3).

ROLE OF THE DENTAL HOME

Just as a multidisciplinary team-based approach is best to monitor comprehensive growth and development of patients with cleft lip and/or cleft palate (CL/P), a primary dental provider, or dental home, is recommended to monitor the dental development of these patients.[6] The role of the dental home is to provide comprehensive care, anticipatory guidance, preventive measures, and treat dental disease based on an individual's unique dental needs.[7] For patients with CL/P, their dental needs are different as they face a childhood with multiple surgical, therapeutic, and dental interventions. These interventions change based on the child's growth and development. Additionally, the child may be seen by the dental home more frequently than their multidisciplinary team; therefore, the role of the dental home is to provide frequent communication with the surgical and therapeutic teams and recommend intervention as needed.

During the primary dentition years (from infancy to 6 years old), the role of the dental home is to oversee presurgical infant orthopedic appliance therapy (PSIO), if applicable, and communicate with the surgeon for surgical timing of lip repair. The dental home should monitor the eruption of the primary dentition, evaluate the patient for dental anomalies commonly found in patients with CL/P (including tooth agenesis, supernumerary teeth, enamel hypoplasia, and tooth-shape anomalies), and provide dietary and disease prevention counseling, including good oral hygiene practices, as patients with CL/P are at an increased risk of dental caries, at a rate that increases between 2 to 6 years.[8,9]

During the mixed dentition years (age 6–12 years old), the role of the dental home is to continue providing disease prevention strategies as dental caries are increased in both primary and permanent dentitions,[8] and to continue to monitor growth and development. At the site of the cleft, a bony deficit may exist, and surgeons may recommend an alveolar bone graft (ABG). The ABG is best performed before the eruption of the maxillary canines, allowing the canines to erupt through the grafted site and carry bone to allow proper bone height at the site(s) of the cleft. Before ABG, maxillary expansion may be required as patients with CL/P may present with a posterior crossbite. Therefore, the role of the dental home in active monitoring of growth and development with frequent clinical and radiographic examination is essential.[3]

During the early permanent dentition years (from age 12 to 18), the role of the dental home remains focused on the prevention and coordination of care. During this stage, the timing of growth is coordinated with comprehensive orthodontics. Once growth has ceased, based on the patient's need, dental implants, orthognathic surgery, postgrowth/surgery orthodontics, and bone grafting may be required. Additionally, if the dental home during childhood has been at a pediatric dentistry office, transition of care and transfer of records to a general dentist is a key component of management for patients with CL/P to allow the continuity of care.

REFERENCES

1. Deeney S, Somme S. Prenatal consultation for foetal anomalies requiring surgery. Women Birth 2016;29(1):e1–7.
2. Vyas T, Gupta P, Kumar S, et al. Cleft of lip and palate: A review. J Fam Med Prim Care 2020;9(6):2621–5.
3. Policy on the Management of Patients with Cleft Lip/Palate and Other Craniofacial Anomalies. Pediatr Dent 2018;40(6):441–2.
4. Grayson BH, Santiago PE, Brecht LE, et al. Presurgical nasoalveolar molding in infants with cleft lip and palate. Cleft Palate Craniofac J 1999;36(6):486–98.
5. Yang S, Stelnicki EJ, Lee MN. Use of nasoalveolar molding appliance to direct growth in newborn patient with complete unilateral cleft lip and palate. Pediatr Dent 2003;25(3):253–6.
6. Definition of Dental Home. Pediatr Dent 2018;40(6):12.
7. Policy on the Dental Home. Pediatr Dent 2018;40(6):29–30.
8. Worth V, Perry R, Ireland T, et al. Are people with an orofacial cleft at a higher risk of dental caries? A systematic review and meta-analysis. Braz Dent J 2017;223(1):37–47.
9. Sunderji S, Acharya B, Flaitz C, et al. Dental Caries Experience in Texan Children with Cleft Lip and Palate. Pediatr Dent 2017;39(5):397–402.

Interdisciplinary Oral Health for Those with Special Health Care Needs

Allen Wong, DDS, EdD, DABSCD*, Lisa Itaya, DDS

KEYWORDS

- Dentistry • Oral health • Special health care needs • Tele-education

KEY POINTS

- There is a need for interdisciplinary care to ensure inclusive quality health care.
- The disparity of care for those with special healthcare needs is greater as there are a lack of trained dental providers.
- New paradigms and technology are needed to help alleviate burdens on the healthcare system.

In order for us to understand our current situation of the oral health condition of those with special needs, we need to review the history of how education was presented and what has been done. The American Dental Association, Commission on Dental Accreditation (CODA) is recognized by the US Department of Education. CODA is responsible for the accreditation of predoctoral dental education programs (leading to the DDS or DMD degree), advanced dental education programs, and allied dental education programs that are fully operational or have attained "Initial Accreditation" status, including programs offered via distance education (https://www2.ed.gov/admins/finaid/accred/accreditation_pg7.html.)

CODA currently defines "Patients with special healthcare needs (SHCN) as patients whose medical, physical, psychological, cognitive or social situations make it necessary to consider a wide range of assessment and care options in order to provide dental treatment. These individuals include, but are not limited to, people with developmental disabilities, cognitive impairment, complex medical problems, significant physical limitations, and the vulnerable elderly."

Associations between dental and chronic systemic diseases were observed frequently in medical research; however, the findings of this research have so far found little relevance in everyday clinical treatment.[1]

University of the Pacific, Arthur A. Dugoni School of Dentistry, 155 Fifth Street, San Francisco, CA 94103, USA
* Corresponding author.
E-mail addresses: allen.wong@aadmd.org; awong@pacific.edu

Dent Clin N Am 66 (2022) 283–291
https://doi.org/10.1016/j.cden.2022.01.006
0011-8532/22/© 2022 Elsevier Inc. All rights reserved.

THE PAST DENTAL FOCUS FOR PATIENTS WITH SPECIAL HEALTH CARE NEEDS

In its accreditation standards published in 2004, the CODA adopted a new standard, to be implemented starting in January 1, 2006, stating that "Graduates must be competent in assessing the treatment needs of patients with special needs." The literature shows that academic dental institutions have a history of underpreparing students to manage the increasing population of individuals with special needs.[2]

Historically, patients with special health care needs (SHCN) were taken care of by those with postdoctoral training, primarily pediatric dentists, hospital dentists, and a minority of general dentists who were mentored or learned along the way. In the 1990s, organizations were formed to support and increase the knowledge of specialized care for those with developmental disabilities. An organization was formed with 3 groups having distinct interests: The American Association of Hospital Dentists, American Society of Geriatric Dentistry, and Academy of Dentistry for Persons with Disabilities. The 3 organizations created the Federation of Special Care Organizations in Dentistry in 1997 and now is known as Special Care Dentistry Association (SCDA) with the same 3 groups known as Councils. The SCDA has annual meetings that promote quality care for those individuals with SHCN with an emphasis in postdoctoral education in clinics, hospitals, and dental schools. The organization supplemented not only what was missing from predoctoral education but also supported training for those interested in learning more about special needs dentistry.

As the population of SHCN increased in numbers through the years, so did their lifespan. In the 1950s, the average lifespan of a person with intellectual and developmental disabilities (IDD) was about 30 years. Now their lifespan is closer to 60 years and they are facing the similar aging comorbid health concerns.

Pediatric dentists are no longer able to provide continuing treatment to an aging patient with comorbidities. Pediatric dentists were reminded of their age-defined specialty in 2000 and encouraged to transition their adult patients to the general dentist.

In 2012, a 10-year retrospective study at the University of the Pacific Arthur A. Dugoni School of Dentistry concluded that the predoctoral and postdoctoral experiences of treating special needs populations seem to correlate to the graduates' practice settings and patient populations. General dentists who did not have a postdoctoral residency experience were less likely to treat patients with SHCN. Continuing education programs were scarce in the area of special needs dentistry for the adult population.[3]

The problem, then and now, is clear: There are fewer providers of dentistry for special needs adults in spite of a large workforce due to lack of trained individuals at the predoctoral and postdoctoral levels. And more importantly, if a person receives education and clinical experiences, then they are more likely to treat this population.

Special Olympics is an organization that focused on the needs of those with IDD since the 1950s with an emphasis on sports. It was the unfortunate dental crisis of Rosemary Kennedy that the founder Eunice Kennedy Shriver (Rosemary's sister) brought great attention to the challenges of adequate and appropriate access to dental care for those with IDD. The situation gave rise to the attention of not only the lack of access but also the disparity of care. Eunice Kennedy Shriver convinced Dr Steve Perlman, the dentist who treated Rosemary, to help her with creating change in the system. Dr Perlman knew that to create change data were needed. He collaborated with the CDC to create a screening tool to capture information from the Special Olympics athletes. In gathering data, it was realized that in addition to oral health disparities, other health concerns existed as well.

The "Surgeon General's Oral Health Report" in 2017 concluded that although common dental diseases are preventable, many people face barriers, sometimes insurmountable, that prevent their access to oral health care. The report outlined a collaborative National Oral Health Plan that is all inclusive and wide ranging in its approach to reducing oral health disparities. Furthermore, it emphasized the importance of focusing on people at the highest risk for specific oral diseases and improving access to existing care. One approach involved making dental insurance available to all Americans.[4]

The Yale Report "The Health Status and Needs of Individuals with Mental Retardation (past accepted terminology)" published on September 15, 2000, identified disparity of care in those with IDD.

Special Olympics was able to help encourage a health summit to discuss the disparities of care before a subcommittee of the US Senate Committee of Appropriations Summit for the first session of a special hearing in Anchorage, Alaska, March 5, 2001. Surgeon General David Satcher hosted his conference on "Health Disparities and Mental Retardation" in December 2001 to acknowledge the disparity of health care and the emphasis that oral health is part of overall health. It was this impetus that led to the formation of the American Academy of Developmental Medicine and Dentistry and the start of a change in ADA CODA Accreditation Standard 2.24. It was a step in the right direction but did not specifically address IDD populations and left SHCNs to be interpreted by institutions. Some institutions defined SHCNs as medically compromised only.

Special Olympics Health disciplines were formed to gather data of those disparities. The disciplines of optometry, audiology, physical therapy, podiatry, nutrition, and mental health created educational and screening tools to help improve our understanding of those disparities as well. Special Olympics realized that for an athlete to reach their sports potential, they needed to be healthy and have quality equitable health care.

In the mid-1990s, the Institute of Medicine (IOM) was asked to study dental education and its direction. There were some recognized barriers identified. IOM published "Dental Education at the Crossroad: Challenges and Change," which focused on the challenges of preparing the dental professional from a retrospective look after the first 150 years of dental education. The new report (1995) from the IOM underscored the need for changes in dental education to prepare for a future that would be, in many important ways, quite different from the past.[5]

Dental education was taught in discipline-specific silos each with their own focus in educating the safe beginning practitioner. Most dental schools screened for patients who were relatively healthy. Patients with significant medical concerns such as radiation therapy, organ transplants, and cardiac conditions were mostly cared for in the private sector or postdoctoral general dentistry (Advanced Education in General Dentsitry (AEGD)/General Practice Residency (GPR)) programs. Very few dental schools until recently had undergraduate special care clinics, whereas the rest depended on didactic lectures to prepare the new clinician.

For the profession to advance, every dental school must play a role in establishing a culture that attaches value to research/discovery, evidence-based practice, and the application of new knowledge/technologies to patient care.[6]

We hope to focus on providing care for all patients safely and not just the healthier ones.

We have been trying for the past couple of decades to address the issues of care through the lens of the "triple aim": improving the patient experience, improving the health of the population, and reducing the cost of healthcare.. Recently, another aim has been identified: lower burnout from providers. As it is burdensome to work in silos, an improved paradigm should be considered.

The time is ripe for institutional programming to create and foster the personal tools needed to prevent burnout and its sequelae with the goal of maintaining the dental workforce and expanding the providers who can treat the special care patient population.[7] If we do not pay attention to provider self-care, we will certainly have a shortage of experienced providers for the growing population.

THE FUTURE ATTENTION FOR SPECIAL HEALTH CARE NEEDS PROVIDERS

The American Dental Association with the encouragement of the American Academy of Developmental Medicine and Dentistry (AADMD) and the National Disability Council (NCD) re-evaluated and revised the ethical consideration of those with IDD and the dental code of ethics. The CODA had meetings with the communities of interest and in 2019 revised the standards for dental education to include an emphasis on people with special health care needs. Instead of just "assessing the needs," there is now a required active component in managing the treatment of special care patients, as well as the appropriate language to use when communicating to and about these patients. It reads (changes in *bold*):

> • *Accreditation Standards for Dental Education Programs, Standard 2-25 "Graduates must be competent in assessing **and managing** the treatment ~~needs~~ of patients with special needs." The intent statement was also changed – "… The assessment should emphasize the importance of non-dental considerations **including the use of respectful nomenclature and supported decision making**….**and providing services or referral as appropriate**. (CODA Standard 2–25, 2019)*

As we look forward to treating the whole person with interdisciplinary and intradisciplinary approaches, we need to look beyond the silos and create a bigger tent approach. Oral care providers not only become excellent technicians in restoring the function of teeth but also will be experts in risk assessments of dental caries and periodontal disease. Recognizing comprehensive needs means more than teeth and gums; it is the patient's whole health we intend to improve with equitable care. Many of these disparity considerations parallel those of adults who have lived with developmental disabilities over a lifetime, and similar prevention principles can be applied. Systemic diseases, conditions, and their treatments can pose significant risks to oral health, thus requiring prevention, treatment, and advocacy for oral health care as integral to chronic disease management.[8]

The pandemic years made us focus on some of the glaring disparities and taught us to use technologies and systems more efficiently. We were able to expand our traditional offices and clinics into virtual offices and clinics. We were able to use technology to help educate and bring access to our patients who could not make appointments due to physical or psychosocial reasons. While telemedicine has been adopted and is used increasingly in patient care, the dental profession is still in the relatively early stages of using technology for teledentistry. The number of patients with intellectual and developmental disabilities is increasing in number and complexity, calling for new approaches to assist with access to care.[9]

We have learned that health care students want to learn how to care for those with IDD and medical compromise through curriculum initiatives. Student chapters of

AADMD/SCDA are forming and increasing awareness in their dental/medical/health care schools and clinics nationwide.

Collaboration and innovation within the oral health disciplines as well as the supporting medical, social, and allied health fields are creating an atmosphere of true comprehensive health care spirit.

Models of telehealth and tele-education help promote the idea of integrated health systems.

TELEHEALTH: TELEMEDICINE, TELEDENTISTRY, TELECONSULTATION, TELE-EDUCATION
Models of Telehealth

Telemedicine has been around since 1974 with steady expansion in the 1990s and an explosion in the 2010 decade especially during the pandemic era from 2019 until now.

Bringing information and experience to those who could not get those resources made sense. Barriers such as encryption and privacy of information were later addressed using enhanced information systems. The pandemic has helped those who were homebound or with limited access to health care to finally get some consultation in the convenience of their homes.

Importantly, clinicians were recognized and compensated for their time thus making the experience more worthwhile, safe, and efficient. There is still the concern of "practicing within borders and licensing," but even those issues are being discussed as governmental agencies and insurance providers are seeking to improve health care systems.

Most medical telehealth are consultations and less dependent on physical contact as opposed to oral health. Both fields require certain "physical assessments," but there are more limitations to the utilization of teledentistry, as dental procedures are mostly "hands on."

Teledentistry has been in the literature since the mid-1990s and mostly for transferring information such as dental records (pictures, charting, and radiographs) rather than actual dental care.

The way that dentistry can effectively use "teledentistry" is in the intake process when getting acquainted with the patient and caregiver.

Technology has allowed us to provide a friendly smile and maskless initial interaction. A true underappreciated use of teledentistry is the area of oral health counseling such as eating habits, nutrition, sleep, and proper oral care techniques.

Virtual Dental Home (VDH) was founded in 2012 by Dr Paul Glassman at the University of the Pacific Arthur A. Dugoni School of Dentistry. The concept was to reach those with difficulties obtaining oral health services. These new methods include delivering oral health services in nontraditional settings, using nondental professionals, expanding roles for existing dental professionals and new types of dental professionals, and incorporating telehealth technologies.[10]

With all new programs, there were advantages and criticisms. A major criticism was that the VDH not only lacked the attributes of a dental home but also had not been shown to be as efficient and effective as traditional programs staffed by dental hygienists and dental therapists.[11]

On a more positive note, it increased awareness to those with challenges in access to care and incorporated the dental team in creative models.

Teleconsultation

Distance consultation is a useful resource for improving accessibility, as well as leading to more physical consultation time; it has also demonstrated that it is capable of solving problems of different kinds and in different age groups.[12] A novel model of care for those with IDD is based on Ruth Ryan's model of whole person assessment.

TACT (Telemedicine Assessment Consultation Team) in Northern California was piloted in the late 1990s and is still active today. TACT is a concentrated team of health care professionals with special experiences and skillsets that consults from a distance with a local health team that works with the patient. The specialized health care team conducts a very comprehensive meeting. The patient is present and in control of the meeting. In the TACT group, each health care consultant is provided a detailed report of the patient's entire health record, given time to review the records, and then meets via videoconference with the patient and the patient's local health team. The consultants are paid for their time to prepare for and participate in the videoconference and to provide a final report. The live interaction allows the patient to ask questions and respond naturally as well as behave naturally in their nonthreatening environment. The consultation team members are free to ask questions within and outside their specialties, thus improving the consultant's knowledge in various areas of medicine.

The cost of the medical assessments is promptly recovered in a variety of savings to systems. Comprehensive medical assessment discloses increased medical comorbidities in persons with mental retardation (the mental retardation term is now referred to as intellectual disability referred for psychiatric evaluation). Comprehensive treatment based on the assessment findings seems to be associated with better clinical outcomes and cost savings to systems.[13]

Tele-education in dentistry is a concept that was implemented out of necessity during the pandemic era. Suddenly, those with IDD who participated with Special Olympic sporting events were prohibited from in-person competitions and practice. Fitness was the focal point for the organization initially until health concerns of individuals were brought to the forefront in the late 1990s as previously mentioned. More importantly, routine oral evaluations, screenings, and oral hygiene instructions at events were not available. There was discussion from Special Olympics International of using teledentistry to bridge the gap of in-person screenings. After careful consideration, the legal aspect of performing teledentistry without a dental home and territorial licensure (state and regional Boards) became a factor. The solution lay in an approach to improve health by improving self-awareness through guided interactions using PowerPoint questions and facilitation.

The program "Virtual Special Smiles Self-Assessment for Special Olympics Athletes" was created and adapted to not only Special Olympics in the United States but also international athletes. The program is universal in its information to improve oral health awareness and is offered to non-Special Olympics groups as well. The PowerPoint presentation has an accompanying guide for use and is downloadable from the Special Olympics Web site for Virtual Special Smiles (https://resources.specialolympics.org/health/special-smiles).

How it works
A group of Special Olympics participants are invited to the interactive program. Facilitators are chosen and invited to participate. Because it is education, health care students can participate and be mentored by a licensed dentist. There is no group "size restriction" other than the limits of the virtual conferencing software.

The Virtual Smiles program is a series of 30 PowerPoint slides that asks questions of the audience and offers a poll to record the results in a virtual conference meeting format. Each question is followed with an answer to reinforce knowledge or teach new knowledge by explaining the "why" of the question to participants. Topics covered are demographics, dental habits, teeth, gums, hydration, oral trauma, and dental urgencies. The goal is to collect relevant data and allow the participant to become more self-aware and self-determined to seek help if needed. After the question session, there is a facilitator wrap up to answer any questions. For larger groups, there are breakout rooms of up to 10 participants to 1 oral health care provider to make the event more personal. At the end of a 10-minute question session, the breakout group returns to a main group.

Finally, there is a question to the participants asking if they would like a private tele-dentistry visit. The host of the event is able to see if any "urgent responses" are reported and would get followed up.

FUTURE OF COLLABORATION

Oral health prevention is not limited to dentists, hygienists, and therapists alone. We need to collaborate with every entity involved with the care of a person. Many patients with SHCN have comorbid health conditions, physical challenges, and diagnostic overshadowing. Diagnostic overshadowing can be described as a concept whereby a health care professional mistakenly attributes symptoms of physical ill health to either a mental health or behavioral problem, or as being inherent in the person's disability; this can lead to a failure to diagnose and treat appropriately. Although widely discussed in medicine, this issue has not been previously highlighted in the dental specialty, yet it can lead to significantly detrimental general and oral health outcomes for vulnerable patients.[14]

Diagnostic overshadowing has led to unnecessary pain, overprescription of medications, health complications, and premature tooth loss.

As oral health educators, we need to educate those who support the individuals that need assistance. A new paradigm in understanding and educating dental and periodontal risks to those not directly in dental care professions is equally important as learning how to treat the disease.

All health professionals and support providers should be aware of mitigating risks in oral health. Those that prescribe medications should be aware of their effects to the oral protective mechanism, saliva. Patients with SHCN have the highest dental caries risk and periodontal problems. Oral care for those with higher risks is more than just about brushing and flossing when possible. It is about preventing the demineralization of teeth in an acidic environment.

Most medications have side effects that can affect and impair the salivary quality and quantity, which in turn increases the risk for dental caries, stomatitis, gastric reflux, and xerostomia.

Medication-induced xerostomia and hyposalivation will increasingly become oral health issues for older and geriatric patients because of the likely high prevalence of medication intake and polypharmacy, with complex negative conditions of dysphagia, caries incidence, malnutrition, and diminished quality of life. All health care professionals are encouraged to investigate dry mouth symptoms among their patients, because diagnosis can easily be performed within daily clinical practice.[15]

Dental providers can educate medical and nursing providers in recognizing xerostomic conditions and risks, as well as train them (depending on geographic licensure limitations) in the applications of preventative therapy like fluoride varnish.

The person with or without disability or health care needs may have oral changes from both external (foods, drinks) and internal (gastric reflux, hyposalivation, hypo salivary gland function) influences. Add the limitation of physical dexterity to properly clean all teeth surfaces, challenges of accessing health care at proper intervals can lead to uncontrolled dental disease.

Proper risk interval dental visits for prevention cannot be overstated. Currently, recall (recare) intervals are based on a model of average healthy populations. For many, this may be effective.

A risk-based recall approach should mitigate the disease through chemotherapeutic agents to arrest or prevent the dental disease from progressing. Those who have a higher risk for a disease should be seen more frequently for prevention therapy.

A collaborative and integrated interdisciplinary approach can maximize both the health of the patient and underscore the quadruple aim for oral health. Nontraditional integration of nurses, physicians, behaviorists, nutritionists, occupational and physical therapists, direct support professionals, social services, insurance industry, advocates, self-advocates, and other associated organizations into dental education could also be valuable.

Not addressing the dental disease and prevention aspect leads to loss of teeth, loss of life, and added costs. Hospital dentistry should always be a last resort to care.

Hospital dentistry is one of the most expensive routes to treating a person, but if we are to invest in such care, we ought to consider the most efficient manner. If a person is uncooperative to receive dental care in a routine setting and needs general anesthesia, the attempt to maximize that procedure should be investigated. The patient's primary care provider should be consulted to orchestrate a comprehensive evaluation of the patient.

We should consider appropriate and needed tests and medical services during the procedure, if possible, for example, additional blood work, electrocardiography, echocardiography, medication therapeutic levels, eye examination, ear examination, Papanicolaou test, podiatric treatment, chest or skull radiographs, or biopsies to name some.

If properly and collaboratively planned, concerted care can occur.

With the increased emphasis in dental education by its accrediting body (CODA) in the area of SHCN management and treatment, a more prepared workforce will be able to provide care, and we look forward to a brighter and healthier future for all our patients.

For those interested in resources in SHCN, here are some references:

American Academy of Developmental Medicine and Dentistry (AADMD) aadmd.org.

Special Care Dentistry Association (SCDA) scdaonline.org.

American Academy of Pediatric Dentistry aapd.org.

Special Olympics resources

https://resources.specialolympics.org/health/special-smiles.

Special Olympics Caregivers Guide (English and Spanisersions available)

https://media.specialolympics.org/resources/health/disciplines/specialsmiles/Special-Smiles-Caregivers-Guide-English-Feb-2020.pdf?_ga=2.171656224.1247959429.1621276023-604982191.1621276023.

Special Olympics Videos from Athletes (6 videos)

https://resources.specialolympics.org/health/special-smiles/how-to-dental-videos?locale=en&fbclid=IwAR1ZwvmREji2H93abfVUuxZW_narecuZ3Cn1yJtVNO0nlUP1cJI4U6aW5Ng.

CLINICS CARE POINTS

- Recognize the healthcare disparities of the whole person, not just their teeth

- Incorporate prevention strategies, such as caries risk and periodontal risk assessment, to avoid oral disease and hospital dentistry
- If hospital dentistry is needed, consider a comprehensive approach with other medical disciplines
- Become the needed workforce through continuing education
- Learn technology like telehealth to improve access to those who need care

REFERENCES

1. Seitz MW, Haux C, Knaup P, et al. Approach towards an evidence-oriented knowledge and data acquisition for the optimization of interdisciplinary care in dentistry and general medicine. Stud Health Technol Inform 2018;247:671–4. https://www.ncbi.nlm.nih.gov/pubmed/29678045.
2. Clemetson JC, Jones DL, Lacy ES, et al. Preparing dental students to treat patients with special needs: changes in predoctoral education after the revised accreditation standard. J Dent Educ 2012;76(11):1457–65. https://www.ncbi.nlm.nih.gov/pubmed/23144481.
3. Subar P, Chavez EM, Miles J, et al. Pre- and postdoctoral dental education compared to practice patterns in special care dentistry. J Dent Educ 2012;76(12):1623–8. https://www.ncbi.nlm.nih.gov/pubmed/23225681.
4. Satcher D, Nottingham JH. Revisiting oral health in america: a report of the surgeon general. Am J Public Health 2017;107(S1):S32–3.
5. Field MJ, Jeffcoat MK. Dental education at the crossroads: a report by the Institute of Medicine. J Am Dent Assoc 1995;126(2):191–5.
6. Iacopino AM. The influence of "new science" on dental education: current concepts, trends, and models for the future. J Dent Educ 2007;71(4):450–62. https://www.ncbi.nlm.nih.gov/pubmed/17468305.
7. Menzin AW, Kline M, George C, et al. Toward the quadruple aim: impact of a humanistic mentoring program to reduce burnout and foster resilience. Mayo Clin Proc Innov Qual Outcomes 2020;4(5):499–505.
8. Chavez EM, Wong LM, Subar P, et al. Dental care for geriatric and special needs populations. Dent Clin North Am 2018;62(2):245–67.
9. Spivack E. Teledentistry: remote observation of patients with special needs. Gen Dent 2020;68(3):66–70. https://www.ncbi.nlm.nih.gov/pubmed/32348247.
10. Glassman P, Harrington M, Namakian M, et al. The virtual dental home: bringing oral health to vulnerable and underserved populations. J Calif Dent Assoc 2012;40(7):569–77. https://www.ncbi.nlm.nih.gov/pubmed/22916378.
11. Friedman JW, Nash DA, Mathu-Muju KR. The virtual dental home: a critique. J Public Health Dent 2017;77(4):302–7.
12. de la Fuente Ballesteros SL, Garcia Granja N, Hernandez Carrasco M, et al. [Telemedicine consultation as a tool to improve the demand for consultation in Primary Care]. Semergen 2018;44(7):458–62.
13. Ryan R, Sunada K. Medical evaluation of persons with mental retardation referred for psychiatric assessment. Gen Hosp Psychiatry 1997;19(4):274–80.
14. Clough S, Handley P. Diagnostic overshadowing in dentistry. Br Dent J 2019;227(4):311–5.
15. Barbe AG. Medication-induced Xerostomia and Hyposalivation in the elderly: culprits, complications, and management. Drugs Aging 2018;35(10):877–85.

Mentorship for the Future Special Care Dentist

Stephen Beetstra, DDS, MHSA

KEYWORDS

- Health care • Medicaid • Mentor • Mentee • Mentorship dyad
- special healthcare needs

KEY POINTS

- Mentorship is vital in creating a competent dental workforce who treat patients with SHCNs.
- Development of Mentorship programs is necessary to maintain a viable provider workforce who treat patients with SHCNs.
- Most mentoring in predoctoral dental education occurs after graduation.
- A concerted effort by academic institutions, professional organizatons, and employers to develop mentorship programs is necessary to secure a long term workforce.

INTRODUCTION

Historically, mentorships and apprenticeships have proven to be vital to the education of competent healthcare clinicians. Up until the Flexner Report in 1910, which states healthcare education must be rooted in science and research, mentorship was the most common training method in becoming a physician or dentist. Mentors play a critical role in the development of professionals by influencing their job satisfaction, career aspirations, and professional identity.[1] As dental school curricula adapt to include an increased volume of science and technology training, dental students no longer receive the same amount of mentoring during their professional education. To offset this reduction in mentoring, a significant portion of mentoring now occurs during optional postgraduate residency training and on-the-job experiences. Although the teaching of science and technology information to students studying to be healthcare providers is important, we should not underestimate the influence an effective mentor has on a mentee's professional career trajectory. Therefore, mentorship should be a priority in the development of dental professionals and emphasized for those who strive to develop the complex skills needed to care for individuals with special health care needs (SHCNs)[2]; this will take a commitment to the relationship by both the mentor and mentee in order to realize the advantages of a mentorship program that benefits all

Dental Program Director, the Nisonger Center, Wexner Medical Center/Ohio State University Dental School, 345 McCampbell Hall, 1581 Dodd Avenue, Columbus, OH 43210, USA
E-mail address: Stephen.beetstra@osumc.edu

Dent Clin N Am 66 (2022) 293–305
https://doi.org/10.1016/j.cden.2021.12.002
0011-8532/22/© 2021 Elsevier Inc. All rights reserved.

stakeholders including providers, patients, and the educational organization. This chapter will examine how the lack of mentoring affects care for special populations, explore the benefits of mentoring programs, explain the cost associated with mentoring, innumerate the characteristics of a good mentor and mentee, provide examples of successful mentorship programs, and highlight personal insights (**Table 1**).

THE ADVANTAGES OF MENTORING HEALTHCARE PROVIDERS WHO CARE FOR PATIENTS WITH SPECIAL HEALTH CARE NEEDS

Treating dental patients with SHCNs is challenging and requires an interdisciplinary approach. Working with people with intellectual or developmental disabilities (IDD) is emotionally consuming, sometimes physically demanding,[3] and cuts across interdisciplinary and interprofessional lines.[4] Most studies that examine this issue come to a similar conclusion in many healthcare fields including medical, dental, and nursing care: there is a lack of exposure to patients with SHCNs during their training, which often adversely affects these clinicians' willingness and ability to manage patients with SHCNs throughout their careers. The absence of a symbiotic mentoring relationship often results in burnout due to the lack of professional support and feelings of isolation. Burnout is defined as a state of emotional, physical, and mental exhaustion caused by excessive and prolonged stress. This stress often results in dental care professionals avoiding employment positions that include care for patients with SHCNs.

Currently, many healthcare workers understand that finding training in the care of individuals with SHCNs most often occurs outside of the traditional learning settings. Providers develop their techniques through observation, trial and error, and on-the-job experience. Acquisition of these skills occurred largely in the workplace rather than as predoctoral dental students or dental hygiene students.[5] As an example, a study concluded physician participants identified themes of "operating without a map," discomfort with patients with an IDD, and a need for more exposure to/experience with people with IDD as important content areas.[6] In the dental profession, this lack of exposure creates feelings of incompetence and an unwillingness of dental care providers to treat patients with SHCNs. These hurdles remain as barriers to providing access to dental care for these populations.[7,8] Finally, in a survey of predoctoral students at the University of Michigan School of Dentistry, most of the respondents did not perceive their undergraduate dental education for the treatment of patients with SHCNs had prepared them to competently provide dental care to the IDD population. The study concluded major efforts should be made to improve dental education in treating these patient populations.[9] Failure to develop competent providers to care for patients with IDD will continue if effective mentorship programs are not provided to dental students, dental hygiene students, and residents of dental training programs; this provides a significant argument as to why the development of mentorship relationships programs is necessary for access and continuity of care for patients with SHCNs.

BENEFITS OF MENTORSHIP PROGRAMS

As explained earlier, most experiential learning in the treatment of the SHCNs population occurs outside the traditional dental or dental hygiene curriculum after graduation. Formal training programs provide the technical knowledge necessary for clinical procedures but often fall short in providing the appropriate guidance in teaching the art of patient management, which requires a significant period of devoted time, practice, and focus to develop. Mentorship programs play a vital role in cultivating patient management skills in a clinical setting. Mentoring is described as a planned relationship between an experienced person and one who has less experience for the purpose of

Table 1

Themes that characterize successful mentoring relationships from a qualitative study on successful and failed mentoring relationships through the departments of medicine at the University of Toronto Faculty of Medicine and the University of California, San Francisco, School of Medicine, 2010.

Successful Characteristics	
Reciprocity	Bidirectional nature of mentoring, including consideration of strategies to make the relationship sustainable and mutually rewarding
Mutual respect	Respect for the mentor and mentee's time, effort, and qualifications
Clear expectations	Expectations of the relationship are outlined at the onset and revisited over time; both mentor and mentee are held accountable to these expectations
Personal connection	Connection between the mentor and mentee
Shared values	Around the mentor's and mentee's approach to research, clinical work, and personal life
Unsuccessful Characteristics	
Lack of commitment	Lack of time committed to the relationship or waning interest over time
Personality differences	Different personal characteristics between the mentor and mentee
Perceived (or real) competition	Overlapping interests may lead to competition; failure to recognize that a mentee's success reflects well on his or her mentor

Data from Cho C, Feldman M, Feldman M. Defining the Ideal Qualities of Mentorship: A Qualitative Analysis of the Characteristics of Outstanding Mentors. The American Journal of Medicine. 2011:124(5):453-458. https://doi.org/10.1016/j.amjmed.2010.12.007.[19]

achieving identified outcomes.[10] The close one-to-one relationship between the mentor and mentee continually develops through a series of stages, eventually resulting in the 2 colleagues working together in a professional relationship based on respect, support, and productivity.[11] So what are the benefits and outcomes of the mentorship relationships, and how can they be quantified? This section will discuss the benefits that occur when successful mentorship programs and relationships are achieved.

Improvement of Job Satisfaction

When strong mentorship relationships are present, job satisfaction for the mentor and mentee improve, which can be manifested in multiple ways. In a study at Boston General by Tracy and colleagues, the mentees responded with the following perspective: those who participated in an effective mentorship program felt more supported by their academic department and gained a greater sense of camaraderie. Most mentees noted the Boston General program's success in the areas of having a role model (83.3%), having increased visibility (82.3%), and having someone to whom they could turn for advice (93.8%).[12] From a mentor's perspective, the relationship can yield significant value; this includes pride in the development of the next generation of healthcare providers, improvement of technical expertise, a renewed sense of purpose, creation of a legacy, a stronger perception of career success, and a sense of belonging.[13] Both mentors and mentees are less likely to exhibit professional burnout or plateau in professional skills when a strong mentor-mentee relationship is present.[13–15] Mentoring sets in motion the process of self-actualization and growth, which leads to an improvement in job satisfaction.[16,17]

Economic Benefits

There are many economic benefits to implementing a successful mentorship program that may affect organizations. With improvement in job satisfaction, there is a lower turnover rate of all employees, not just the providers, which will prevent staff attrition, and the increase in operational cost associated with recruitment and orientation, as well as loss of revenue during periods of time when staff levels fall short. In addition to cost considerations, staff vacancies negatively affect the morale of senior staff who are often asked to work in understaffed circumstances or provide extra shifts. Staff burnout is often the result. Having well-defined and successful mentorship programs enhances productivity, improves efficiency, creates a recruitment advantage, and increases retention of experienced members.[13] Continuous replacement of providers or staff can be catastrophic to the economic position of an organization or private practice. Successful practices often have a history of retention of employees for extended periods of time, which may be created by a formal or informal mentorship program.

Patient Safety

Patient safety is the prevention of harm to patients. Positive clinical outcomes are enhanced by the creation of successful mentorship programs. Having a mentor available to demonstrate, coach, stimulate ideas, and simulate techniques leads to improved job performance, increased confidence of the mentee, enriched patient experiences, and positive treatment outcomes.[15] One view of a positive treatment outcome includes treatment that improves the health status of the patient and creates an environment that is supportive of the patient's psychological, emotional, and physical needs. The provider's ability to care for SHCNs populations also positively affects the overall performance of the healthcare team. For example, if a provider perfects behavior management techniques, support staff stress is decreased, the healthcare team morale is enhanced, and staff turnover decreases. Patients with SHCNs thrive with familiarity, so often their behavior will deteriorate as a result of turnover of healthcare team members. Staff turnover may lead to adverse treatment outcomes because significant behavioral issues may arise with unfamiliar providers and result in reduced patient compliance.

CHARACTERISTICS OF A GOOD MENTOR

It is important to note there is a significant difference between a mentor and a supervisor, and in most cases, they should not be the same individual. A mentor is someone who acts as a guide rather than someone who directs and evaluates a mentee's activities. Mentoring is not intended to replace the important role of the educational director or supervisor, who has the task of overseeing the trainee's or employee's progress with emphasis on assessment and their portfolio. The mentor is there to provide the mentee with additional and more frequent support pertaining to everyday concerns.[11] In a qualitative data study using interviews of junior faculty by Straus, participants stated mentors "need to be guides, be sensitive to the difference between a guide and somebody who forces the student mentee on to a particular path," and mentors "may well offer some advice but recognize that it is only advice, it's not orders." Another participant said, "The most important thing is not trying to solve their problems but to help them find solutions." The roles of a mentor are to assist the mentee in professional development, offer career guidance and emotional support, and advise them on appropriate work/life balance.[18] Teaching mentorship skills for mentees to become future mentors makes mentorship self-sustaining. By encouraging mentors to affect the future of mentorship, the field becomes stronger and increases the impact on academic and healthcare organizations.[19]

Career Guidance

A primary responsibility of a mentor is to provide career guidance. This guidance should include advising, advocating on behalf of the mentee, facilitating access to career opportunities, goal setting, career monitoring, and assisting mentees in navigating opportunities for potential employment.[17] In these areas, it is important the mentor provide emotional support and honest, critical feedback. All mentorship relationships must be built on trust, and strict confidentiality must be maintained. A mentor must be able to balance what would be beneficial to the institution and the mentee while always keeping the best interest of the mentee in mind. A mentor should be forward thinking and spot future opportunities for the mentee that would enhance their career objectives and development. Often supervisors are obligated to keep the best interests of the institution ahead of mentees' interests. This conflict often creates unhealthy mentor/mentee relationships and should be avoided unless a clear delineation of responsibilities of the supervisor and mentor is established.

From personal experience, I was involved in both successful and unsuccessful mentor/mentee relationships with my supervisors. One successful supervisory mentor clearly spoke to the needs of the organization as well as my individual career goals. Often his career advice was different from the position of the organization. In another instance, an assigned supervisory mentor placed his own personal interests above mine, never gave honest or critical feedback, and did not maintain confidentiality. This dynamic created a dysfunctional relationship void of trust, which increased the dysfunction within the academic department. To prevent a conflict of interest in the supervisory dynamic, many successful mentorship programs are interdisciplinary or interdepartmental in nature. This approach allows for a defined manager in their department of employment and encourages mentor relationships with other faculty or professional staff from a variety of disciplines. Dental providers in nonacademic settings who care for patients with SHCNs are at a disadvantage in finding nonsupervisory mentors. Programs tend to be small (1 or 2 providers), and mentor options are often limited. In this situation, it is recommended the mentee use an interdisciplinary mentor, a dental provider outside their organization, or seek a mentor through a professional organization whose membership includes providers with vast experience treating patients with SHCNs. Engaging a mentor who is empathetic to the day-to-day stresses of caring for individuals with SCHNs is vital to the mentee's development.

Emotional Support and Work/Life Balance

Dental providers who care for patients with SHCNs often face significantly more stress than traditional clinicians due to the extensive medical, behavioral, and dental management needed to provide successful oral healthcare. These patient populations are vulnerable, medically complex, elderly, or have intellectual and developmental disabilities (IDD). Providers serving these populations are often asked to provide services in nontraditional dental treatment environments (nursing homes, hospitals, group homes, and so forth). We perform procedures that can be life-threatening to the patient, are always medically necessary, and as a result, may result in adverse outcomes due to pre-existing medical conditions. In this environment, it is necessary to have mentors who can provide guidance and emotional support to junior providers. In order to manage work-related stress, a mentor must demonstrate and model an appropriate work/life balance. Another study by Straus showed if a mentor possessed an appropriate work/life balance, their mentee also demonstrated an improved work/life balance, reduced work-related stress, and a higher level of job satisfaction. It is important for the mentor and mentee to make time for family and friends, hobbies, and for themselves.[17] In addition, Straus's study reported improvements in communication were seen between mentors and mentees when the mentor shared emotions honestly and modeled appropriate ways to handle work-related stress. Having the mentor help identify relevant stressors for the mentee and how it affected their emotional state improved job performance and quality of professional life.[17] It is essential for both the mentor and mentee to take care of their physical, emotional, and mental health to develop a successful mentorship relationship and overall career.[2,16]

Personal Qualities of a Good Mentor

There are certain characteristics associated with effective mentors. The words most commonly used to describe an outstanding mentors' personality include compassionate, enthusiastic, generous, honest, insightful, selfless, and wise. In particular, selflessness was a prevalent description of mentors.[18] Other characteristics identified by Gisbert include altruistic, available, flexible, critical when needed, and the ability to maintain a positive attitude toward failure.[2] Having the ability to put others' needs above your own and be self-aware of your own strengths and weaknesses seems to be vital in becoming a great mentor.

Supports Needed for Creation of Mentors

Successful mentors require intentional training, as well as institutional support in the form of time and monetary resources. Ramani identified 3 domain areas that lead to mentor success.[1]

1. Development: the mentor needs training to enhance their listening and feedback skills, improve their awareness of gender and cultural issues, and develop clear professional boundaries. Gender and cultural issues are major reasons for unsuccessful mentoring relationships, so intensive training in this area is needed to create successful mentors.
2. Recognition: recognition endorses the mentor needs to be acknowledged for their activities, have protected time for mentoring administration, and receive some rewards (financial or nonfinancial) for their activities.
3. Support: mentors need peer support, a mentor themselves, and a mechanism for referral if issues arise within the mentorship relationship. In structured academic mentorship programs, one or more faculty members should be identified as coaches to help mentors navigate difficulties. It is important that the faculty coaches maintain the characteristics of an excellent mentor and adhere to strict confidentiality.

Even though some mentorship relationships occur organically, having these supports and a formalized structure available to mentors increases the likelihood of long-term success.

Many dental professionals whose main area of practice includes providing care for patients with SHCNs possess the characteristics to become good mentors. They often demonstrate the empathy, compassion, and altruism needed to care for this patient population. One challenge in finding effective mentors for those wanting to work with patients with SHCNs is the nationwide shortage of current oral health providers who focus on caring for these populations. Some reasons those with SHCNs are highly underserved is providers' salaries tend to be lower and the actual practice is more physically, intellectually, and emotionally taxing than other areas of dentistry. Almost 100% of the patient population with SHCNs are covered by Medicaid or a Medicaid-managed care programs, so dental reimbursement for this population ranges from 0% to 50% of normal fees if the state of patient residence provides dental benefits for adults. These reimbursement issues limit dental providers' salaries and often prevents practitioners from providing substantial services to these populations due to economic factors. In addition to the economic constraints of treating patients with SHCNs, managing complex behavioral and medical issues is emotionally and intellectually taxing, as well as time consuming, resulting in reduced productivity. It is difficult for many recent graduates to work with populations of patients with SHCNs due to the low compensation and because of student debt acrrued as a result of the increased cost of dental school tuition. This continual cycle of low reimbursement and stress will exacerbate provider shortages for SHCNs population and will create additional scarcities of mentors in the future if left in the current state.

CHARACTERISTICS OF A GOOD MENTEE

The mentor/mentee relationship begins as an unequal power dynamic due to a difference in experience within an organization or profession. In order to have a successful experience, the mentee must be open to advice, as well as be inquisitive and respectful as the process begins. Management research has shown personality characteristics can influence a person's likelihood of receiving effective mentoring. Individuals with good internal control, high self-monitoring skills, and emotional stability were more active in seeking a mentoring relationship, which in turn contributed to receiving effective mentoring and career success.[20] Characteristics of an effective mentee include the following:

- Being receptive to feedback
- Listening actively
- Respecting the mentor's time
- Meeting agreed deadlines
- Taking responsibility for managing the mentor–mentee relationship
- Investing in one's own learning[21]

Mentees who see themselves as future mentors are more successful in their career development, and this may be the result of having a positive mentoring experience early on in their career, which led to improved job satisfaction and performance. As stated earlier, dental providers who choose to serve patients with SHCNs often display positive characteristics to become excellent mentors. Many mentees see themselves as future teachers and choose to work in positions that train students and residents. Once again, educational debt is an issue for mentees. Loan repayment and forgiveness programs need to be expanded to incentivize and allow individuals who choose to care for patients with SHCNs economic relief from their student loan debt burden.

CHARACTERISTICS OF UNSUCCESSFUL MENTOR/MENTEE RELATIONSHIPS

All healthcare studies concerning successful mentor/mentee relationships have a common thread in which the relationship needs to be beneficial to the mentor as well as the mentee. On the other hand, an unsuccessful mentoring relationship can result in anger, isolation, frustration, and low job satisfaction. In fact, an unsuccessful relationship is a lose-lose-lose relationship in that the mentor, the protégé, and the profession at large suffer from its negative effects.[22] Mentorship dyads (a group of 2 people in an interactional mentorship relationship) that are dominated by one individual are unsuccessful and may be detrimental to both the mentor and mentee due to the perception of lack of commitment to the mentoring process. Straus's groundbreaking work identified characteristics of successful and unsuccessful mentoring relationships in an academic health center.[18]

The importance of the initial stage of the mentor/mentee relationship cannot be underestimated. For instance, most mentees like to choose their own mentor. This can create difficulties in training and academic programs because at the start of a new placement, trainees are not familiar with all the possible mentors.[11] If an unproductive or dysfunctional relationship develops, the mentor or mentee should have the opportunity to discontinue the relationship. The major pitfalls of a poor mentor/mentee dyad include incompatibility of the dyad, lack of expertise of the mentor, ineffective communication, inappropriate identification of the objectives, and poorly stated expectations for the relationship.[21] Development of a system/questionnaire/procedure that yields a high degree of functional mentor/mentee dyads in special care dentistry is an area that needs to be researched, developed, and standardized.

Mentoring in the dental workplace has a unique challenge unlike other healthcare settings. Medical providers are predominately hospital-based or colocated in large group practices in which clinical revenues are often consolidated and salaries are based on relative value units and experience. Dentistry traditionally has a business structure in which revenue is generated by an owner operator's clinical practice and the provision of services. Dentists practice in solitary, small group, or corporate practices in which income depends on a provider's individual collections regardless of age or experience. The possible loss of income due to the time commitment involved in working with a mentee often discourages mentoring relationships until the mentor dental provider has met his/her career economic goals, often near or at retirement; this occurs due to the economic necessity of practice transitions to ensure access to care for the current patients of record. The current economic model in dentistry often hampers successful mentoring of new graduates who desire to care for patients with IDD in the private sector. Existing practices with a focus on these populations, in most cases, accept public insurances that have a lower profit margin due to lower reimbursement rates. This economic disadvantage discourages and prohibits effective mentoring opportunities in special care dentistry. To offset this dilemma, it is important for academic and hospital institutions to create dental training programs specifically focused on those with SHCNs that include an emphasis on mentorship. In addition, our professional organizations need to create structured mentorship programs to assist new graduates serving the SHCNs populations.

TYPES OF MENTORSHIP PROGRAMS

There are 2 basic types of mentoring relationships, formal and informal. Both can be highly effective, and both may occur during the course of one's career. The formal program is often structured and regimented, whereas the informal is more fluid. If either of these relationships are successful, the relationship will transform over time from a mentor/mentee to a mutually beneficial peer relationship.

Formal Mentorship Programs

Formal mentorship programs are created and are commonly used in training programs and professional organizations. They may be regimented and almost always have a set duration of time. Often, the mentor is assigned to the mentee. Mentor training and appropriate mentor/mentee pairings provide a greater likelihood for success in formal mentorship programs. Also, many formal programs do not want to show favoritism to their faculty, so many experienced healthcare providers are asked to be a mentor who do not have the skills to be successful in this role.[23] Business and industry have created many types of formal mentorship programs. In healthcare, Ramani and colleagues discussed the types of formal mentorship program used currently.[24] These programs include the following:

- Speed mentoring: in a format similar to speed dating, mentees rotate from possible mentor to mentor and pose individual questions and discuss a variety of issues related to their career goals and interests in order to find a productive mentorship match. This format should be used by our professional organizations at national meetings that have dental members whose practice focus is patients with SHCNs. With so few providers nationwide whose focus is on these populations, it would allow multiple encounters by junior providers to meet and possibly develop a successful mentorship dyad.
  - Benefits: mentees obtain several perspectives in response to their questions.
  - Challenges: follow-up by the participants is difficult due to the limited contact between the mentor and mentee.
- Small group or team mentoring: multiple mentors work with multiple mentees at one time in a group setting; this is often used in academia and clinical training programs when professors have multiple students progressing at different stages of their education in working laboratory or clinical groups. Besides academia or residency programs, this model could be successful for dental providers as a statewide initiative. Less populated states that have fewer providers who care for the patient populations with SHCNs could easily form mentorship groups containing several states in a region. This model would assist new providers in navigating reimbursement and regulatory issues often created at the state level.
  - Benefits: mentees experience multiple perspectives at once and are able to develop multiple relationships with mentors in a compressed timeframe.
  - Challenges: management of difficult group dynamics can become contentious if conflict occurs between mentees, mentees/mentors, or mentors. Also, mentors may lack training in moderating a laboratory/seminar/clinical scenario that includes several mentees at different stages of training. Finally, organizing meetings with multiple participants can be difficult due to varied clinical schedules, time zones or lack of economic resources.
- Micromentoring: this provides frequent brief meetings that are created to discuss narrow topics. For new providers who want to focus on patients with SHCNs in the private sector, this mentorship relationship would be beneficial. Finding an experienced provider to help a new graduate navigate the process of building a practice, understanding the additional regulations that pertain to practicing in nontraditional dental settings, and understanding the models of reimbursement would also be helpful.
  - Benefits: these meetings occur frequently and address follow-up topics to clinical experiences and can be designed to follow a set curriculum.
  - Challenges: miscommunication may occur due to the inability of the mentee to dive deeply into a particular subject area, as the topic is structured and scheduled to be brief.

- Peer mentoring: colleagues at a similar level mentor each other. For dental providers, this may be beneficial to have a peer mentorship dyad in addition to a traditional mentorship dyad. Communication is often easier between individuals going through the same experiences. This type of mentorship has its disadvantages because the mentor lacks experience and institutional memory that are often necessary for success.
  - Benefits: often the 2 individuals are going through shared experiences and have many similarities. Individuals often feel safe when discussing issues with a peer.
  - Challenges: the peers have not developed the skillset for professional development or the institutional history to allow for networking or navigation of institutional systems.
- Reverse mentoring: a junior mentor is assigned to a senior mentee to assist in assimilating new technology. This model is very successful when the junior mentor has skills the senior mentee is missing. Oral healthcare providers use this model successfully in transitioning electronic records and adding digital technology to practice.
  - Benefits: the junior mentor possesses a skill set that benefits the senior mentee in navigating new systems. Sharing this skill set with a senior provider empowers the junior clinician.
  - Challenges: the junior mentor may not have the mentoring skills or is unwilling or uncomfortable to be critical of the senior mentee.
- Situational or functional mentoring: a mentorship program that is developed for a clear program/project with a set start and end date. This type of mentorship program can be beneficial when dealing with a specific issue. In graduate dental training programs, this model is often used when a resident is having difficulty. Often a mentor is assigned by the program director for a defined period of time or until the resident has successfully demonstrated competency.
  - Benefit: the program is easily quantifiable to determine if it is successful or not as seen by a completed project.
  - Challenges: the mentoring relationship may stagnate, and growth does not occur due to the imposed timeline. Long-term relationships rarely develop, as most of the focus was on the project or program and not the relationship itself.
- Virtual mentoring: with the improvement of digital meeting platforms, technology has allowed for mentor/mentee programs to occur without regard to proximity. Our professional organizations must use this model more frequently and effectively. Efforts to develop webinars are valuable educational tools but most commonly do not allow interaction between the expert and the students. I recommend that our professional organizations develop virtual mentorship platforms to develop these relationships.
  - Benefits: mentees now have the ability to develop relationships outside their immediate geographically area, which greatly expands the number of possible mentors. Maintaining these relationships is now possible, as travel is no longer a necessity.
  - Challenges: sometimes without in-person meetings, relationship are not as robust and some nonverbal communication may be lost. As with most technology, security issues may arise, and care must be taken to remain compliant with regulations.

Informal Mentorship Programs

Informal mentoring relationships usually occur organically over time and often have no set duration. In most, but not all, cases, it is the mentee who approaches the mentor. Some of these mentorship dyads last years or decades and continue due to the creation of a strong interpersonal relationship, the feelings of respect, and the friendship that is created between the mentor and mentee. In informal mentoring relationships, the mentee assumes the mentor chooses to participate by choice and not by obligation. Informal mentors typically have stronger communication skills than formal mentors as perceived by the mentee.[22] The hope is long-term professional networks are developed that allow for the sharing of professional information and collegial support throughout the entirety of a clinician's career. Individuals may often have multiple mentors throughout their career or simultaneously, and some may be outside their own profession. Often interdisciplinary mentorships are successful due to the transferability of skills, institutional knowledge, compatibility of personalities, and the avoidance of the supervisor/employee relationship. Fortunately for me, I am involved in an informal mentorship dyad that has lasted more than 20 years. Over the years, the power dynamic has shifted from a mentor/mentee to a peer relationship. I personally benefitted from this relationship, which helped me to hone my clinical skills, set career goals, and to think holistically about issues that affect the dental profession, oral health professionals, and patient populations I serve.

PREDOCTORAL MENTORSHIP CONSIDERATIONS

Mentoring is a tool that can lead to improved patient safety, provider satisfaction, professional development, and may even lead to cost savings to organizations and practices. Today, most mentoring occurs after graduation, in residency training programs and on the job. The creation of mentorship programs early in training is especially important for providers caring for patients with SHCNs due to the limited exposure new dental graduates receive in their training with these populations. It will take creative thinking and prioritizing mentorship at the predoctoral dental educational level to change this dynamic. The following is list of priorities that should be implemented during the final 2 years of predoctoral education to increase students' exposure to the care of SCHNs patient populations:

- The implementation of extended clinical rotations in geriatric dentistry, dentistry for medically complex patients including oral medicine, and dentistry for IDD populations for students who show interest in working with these groups.
- The standardization of mentorship requirements in the predoctoral educational setting to include working with patients with SHCNs.
- Mentorship training programs for faculty should be funded and developed in oral health education settings.
- Professional oral health organizations should create mentoring registries where mentees are able to view profiles of potential mentors and choose an appropriate pairing for their career goals.

SUMMARY

Whether it is formal or informal, organizations and providers overwhelmingly agree successful mentorship programs and relationships improve patient, staff, and provider satisfaction and performance, as well as reduce staff turnover. In addition, the organization must value the mentorship process by setting aside time and resources for both the mentor and mentee to participate. A successful mentorship relationship increases patient safety and allows clinicians to feel competent in their patient management skills.

The creation of effective mentors will require the commitment of both academic and professional dental organizations to training, supporting, and recognizing excellence in mentor development. This commitment should yield an increase in new dental providers who feel confident in providing oral healthcare services to individuals with SHCNs. With faculty and clinicians who excel at mentoring in special care dentistry, the gap in access to oral healthcare for this underserved population should begin to decrease, ensuring access to dental services for individuals with SCHNs in the future.

Unfortunately, dentistry seems to lag behind other healthcare professions in the creation of mentorship programs. The profession's business model and clinical structures are often contradictory to the creation of programs due to the impact on the mentor's income. To eliminate this barrier, organized dentistry, dental education (predoctoral and graduate), and interdisciplinary organizations need to take a larger role in creating mentorship programs for providers who care for patients with SCHNs. With the improvement in technology, proximity is no longer necessary for the implementation and maintenance of these programs. If successful, the creation of mentorship programs will secure access to dental care for patients with SHCNs by assisting in training the next generation of special care dental professionals.

DISCLOSURE

A special thanks to Joan Beetstra, MS SLP-CCC and Edward Perlow, DDS for their input into this chapter.

REFERENCES

1. Ramani S, Gruppen L, Krajic Kachur E. Twelve tips for developing effective mentors. Med Teach 2006;28(5):404–8.
2. Gisbert JP. La relación mentor-aprendiz en medicina. Gastroenterología y Hepatología. 2017;40(1):48–57.
3. Skirrow P, Hatton C. 'Burnout' amongst direct care workers in services for adults with intellectual disabilities: a systematic review of research findings and initial normative data. J Appl Res Intellect Disabilities 2007;20:131–44.
4. Finkelstein A, Bachner YG, Greenberger C, et al. Correlates of burnout among professionals working with people with intellectual and developmental disabilities. J Intellect Disabil Res 2018;62:864–74.
5. Mac Giolla Phadraig C, Griffiths C, McCallion P, et al. How dentists learn behaviour support skills for adults with intellectual developmental disorders: A qualitative analysis. Eur J Dent Educ 2020;24:535–41.
6. Wilkinson J, Dreyfus D, Cerreto M, et al. "Sometimes I Feel Overwhelmed": Educational Needs of Family Physicians Caring for People with Intellectual Disability. Intellect Dev Disabil 2012;50(3):243–50.
7. Steinberg BJ. Issues and challenges in special care dentistry. J Dent Educ 2005; 69(3):323–4.
8. Kleinert HL, Sanders C, Mink J, et al. Improving Student Dentist Competencies and Perception of Difficulty in Delivering Care to Children with Developmental Disabilities Using a Virtual Patient Module. J Dent Educ 2007;71:279–86.
9. Dao LP, Zwetchkenbaum S, Inglehart MR. General Dentists and Special Needs Patients: Does Dental Education Matter? J Dent Educ 2005;69:1107–15.
10. Dorsey L, Baker C. Mentoring Undergraduate Nursing Students. Nurse Educ 2004;29(6):260–5.

11. Cowan F, Flint S. The importance of mentoring for junior doctors. BMJ 2012;345: e7813.

12. Tracy EE, Jagsi R, Starr R, et al. Outcomes of a pilot faculty mentoring program. Am J Obstet Gynecol 2004;191(6):1846–50. https://doi.org/10.1016/j.ajog.2004. 08.002.

13. Coates WC. Being a Mentor: What's in It for Me? Acad Emerg Med 2012;19:92–7.

14. Sambunjak D, Straus SE, Marušić A. Mentoring in Academic Medicine: A Systematic Review. JAMA 2006;296(9):1103–15. https://doi.org/10.1001/jama.296.9. 1103.

15. Burke RJ, McKeen CA, McKenna C. Benefits of Mentoring in Organizations: The Mentor's Perspective. J Managerial Psychol 1994;9(3):23–32.

16. Crowe SE. Personal perspectives on mentoring. Gastroenterology 2013;144: 488–91.

17. Klein E, Dickenson-Hazard N. "The Spirit of Mentoring," Reflections on Nursing Leadership. Sigma Theta Tau Int 2000;3:18–22.

18. Straus SE, Johnson MO, Marquez C, et al. Characteristics of successful and failed mentoring relationships: a qualitative study across two academic health centers. Acad Med 2013;88(1):82–9.

19. Cho C, Feldman M, Feldman M. Defining the Ideal Qualities of Mentorship: A Qualitative Analysis of the Characteristics of Outstanding Mentors. Am J Med 2011;124(5):453–8.

20. Turban DB, Dougherty TW. Role of protégé personality in receipt of mentoring and career success. Acad Manage J 1994;37:688–702.

21. Straus SE, Chatur F, Taylor M. Issues in the mentor–mentee relationship in academic medicine: a qualitative study. Acad Med 2009;84:135–9.

22. Barker ER. Mentoring—A complex relationship. J Am Acad Nurse Pract 2006;18: 56–61.

23. Ragins BR, Cotton JL. Mentor functions and outcomes: A comparison of men and women in formal and informal mentoring relationships. J Appl Psychol 1999; 84(4):529–50.

24. Ramani S, Thampy H, McKimm J, et al. Twelve tips for organizing speed mentoring events for healthcare professionals at small or large-scale venues. Med Teach 2020;42(12):1322–9.

Moving?

Make sure your subscription moves with you!

To notify us of your new address, find your **Clinics Account Number** (located on your mailing label above your name), and contact customer service at:

Email: journalscustomerservice-usa@elsevier.com

800-654-2452 (subscribers in the U.S. & Canada)
314-447-8871 (subscribers outside of the U.S. & Canada)

Fax number: 314-447-8029

Elsevier Health Sciences Division
Subscription Customer Service
3251 Riverport Lane
Maryland Heights, MO 63043

*To ensure uninterrupted delivery of your subscription, please notify us at least 4 weeks in advance of move.